AF743244

THE GUT MICROBIOME - IMPLICATIONS FOR HUMAN DISEASE

Edited by **Gyula Mozsik**

The Gut Microbiome - Implications for Human Disease
http://dx.doi.org/10.5772/61423
Edited by Gyula Mozsik

Contributors

Suzanne L Ishaq, André-Denis Wright, Peter Moses, Kimberly Cheng, Hein Min Tun, Frederick Leung, Ding-You Li, Min Yang, Sitang Gong, Shui Ye, Sonia Bhardwaj, Zhiheng Pei, Richard Hickman, Maryem Hussein

Published by InTech

Janeza Trdine 9, 51000 Rijeka, Croatia

© The Editor(s) and the Author(s) 2016

The moral rights of the editor(s) and the author(s) have been asserted.
All rights to the book as a whole are reserved by InTech. The book as a whole (compilation) cannot be reproduced, distributed or used for commercial or non-commercial purposes without InTech's written permission. Enquiries concerning the use of the book should be directed to InTech's rights and permissions department (permissions@intechopen.com).
Violations are liable to prosecution under the governing Copyright Law.

(cc) BY

Individual chapters of this publication are distributed under the terms of the Creative Commons Attribution 3.0 Unported License which permits commercial use, distribution and reproduction of the individual chapters, provided the original author(s) and source publication are appropriately acknowledged. More details and guidelines concerning content reuse and adaptation can be found at http://www.intechopen.com/copyright-policy.html.

Notice

Statements and opinions expressed in the chapters are these of the individual contributors and not necessarily those of the editors or publisher. No responsibility is accepted for the accuracy of information contained in the published chapters. The publisher assumes no responsibility for any damage or injury to persons or property arising out of the use of any materials, instructions, methods or ideas contained in the book.

Publishing Process Manager Romina Rovan

Technical Editor SPi Global

Cover InTech Design team

First published November, 2016

Printed in Croatia

Additional hard copies can be obtained from orders@intechopen.com

The Gut Microbiome - Implications for Human Disease, Edited by Gyula Mozsik

p. cm.

Print ISBN 978-953-51-2750-5
Online ISBN 978-953-51-2751-2

We are IntechOpen, the world's leading publisher of Open Access books

Built by scientists, for scientists

3,500+
Open access books available

111,000+
International authors and editors

115M+
Downloads

151
Countries delivered to

Our authors are among the
Top 1%
most cited scientists

12.2%
Contributors from top 500 universities

WEB OF SCIENCE™

Selection of our books indexed in the Book Citation Index in Web of Science™ Core Collection (BKCI)

Interested in publishing with us?
Contact book.department@intechopen.com

Numbers displayed above are based on latest data collected.
For more information visit www.intechopen.com

For EU product safety concerns:
IN TECH d.o.o., Prolaz Marije Krucifikse Kozulić 3, 51000 Rijeka, Croatia,
info@intechopen.com or visit our website at intechopen.com.

Meet the editor

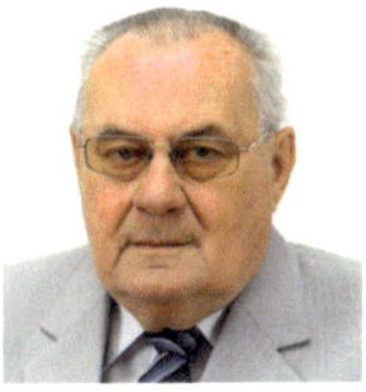

Gyula Mozsik, MD, PhD, ScD (med), is a professor emeritus of medicine at the First Department of Medicine, University of Pécs, Hungary. He was the head of this department from 1993 to 2003. His specialization includes internal medicine, gastroenterology, and clinical pharmacology. His research fields are biochemical pharmacological studies in the gastrointestinal tract, experimental and clinical gastroenterology, clinical pharmacology, experimental and clinical nutrition and dietetics, innovative pharmacological and nutritional (dietetical) researches, and new drug and food productions. He published more than 350 papers in peer-reviewed journals and 19 monographs and edited 30 books. He received André Robert award from the International Union of Pharmacology, Gastrointestinal Section (2014). Fourteen of his students were appointed as full university professors in Cuba, Egypt, and Hungary.

Contents

Preface

The book entitled *The Gut Microbiome—Implications for Human Disease* represents a view in absolutely new and interdisciplinary fields of medical research. To understand the details of these scientific problems in medicine, it is necessary to give some general information from previous decades of medical sciences.

From the 1970s, the medical practice was more inclined to "problem-orientated medicine." The key point was to establish the correct diagnosis in medical practice respecting the most medically effective and economically basic laws. After this period (from the 1980s), the "evidence-based medicine" terminology appeared in different branches of medical sciences to describe the effects of different therapeutic activities. This method is still present in the current medical practice.

Interesting is the fact that the first steps of "evidence-based medicine" appeared earlier in general practice, when physicians wanted to know more about their medical activities, and surprisingly these studies led us to establish the human clinical pharmacology.

The efficiency of pharmacological treatments was critically evaluated in medical treatment. Probably, peptic ulcer disease was the first field in this international process. Objective clinical pharmacological methods were created in these years, and these methods offered objective results on absorption, metabolism, and excretion of different clinically applied drugs. These results clearly indicated that different drugs were not able to be absorbed in the gastrointestinal tract. After these unsuccessful medical therapies, surgical interventions were practiced in unhealed patients (Mózsik Gy., Szabo I.L. (2016) Membrane-Bound ATP-Dependent Energy Systems and Gastrointestinal Mucosa Damage and Protection. InTech, Rijeka, DOI: 10.5772/60095).

This clinical pharmacological research line produced many multiclinical, randomized perspectives and multicentric studies all over the world (including many meta-analyses).

In our days, we have to learn how many basic and clinical pharmacological studies were carried out in the last decades (of course, many medical practices changed after 2005, when Marshall and Warren received the Nobel Prize for the *Helicobacter* pylori research).

Our knowledge from nutrition and especially from dietetics was very limited in terms of medical information. We do not have enough knowledge on food preparation, on the extent of food intake, and also on details of mechanisms of digestion (which absolutely would be necessary and important to understand the details of human nutrition and dietetic therapeutics).

Surprisingly clinical pharmacological methodologies entered the clinical practice earlier than the necessary methods in the field of clinical nutrition and dietetics. From the last century and up to our days, we only had statistical data on food consumption including the different laboratory examinations on (patients') health from medical services.

There are contradictions between differences of methodologies and requirements of clinical pharmacology and clinical nutrition (dietetics). When talking about drugs, the quantiles detected are small. Examining from a chemical perspective, xenobiotics and their measuring methods are specific to xenobiotics. Isotopic methods can be used to measure whole drugs and their metabolites, meanwhile the methods used in nutrition measure the components that are in our bodies; however, whole foods cannot be measured (exception in some special diseases). Generally, it can be recognized that the methodologies of human clinical nutrition and dietetics are more complicated than those of human clinical pharmacology (from a practical point of view, it is important to note that studies about gastrointestinal tract are an essential part of clinical nutrition and dietetics).

Clinical pharmacology and clinical nutrition studies have to carry out observations from phase I to phase IV (which actually equal to each other). We earlier established the methodology of human phase I (Mózsik Gy., Figler M. (2005): Metabolic Ward in Human Clinical Nutrition and Dietetics. Research Signpost, Kerala).

It has to be said that for the realization of these types of special departments, many governmental decisions are necessary for innovative research in the abovementioned fields.

Here is a list of some important events in the last decades of medical life:

1. Trowell (1960–1978) discovered and introduced the terminology of "noninfective population diseases." The recognition of this very important discovery that affects a large portion of the world's population is relevant, and it helps solve many problems with the so-called different "causative and preventive factors" in medical practice, in agriculture, in the food industry and processing, and in medical research.

2. In the years 1971–1980, there was a decrease of intake of dietary fibers. Special researches about dietary fibers significantly changed the food industry practices aimed at increasing dietary fiber intakes through different foods. In those years, it was clear that the contents and species of gut bacterial flora changed significantly depending on the intake of dietary fibers. However at that time, there were no internationally acclaimed institutes in this field to scientifically clarify the changes in the gut bacterial flora.

3. The nutritional habits of different nations changed significantly in the last decades, which produced a wide scale of diseases and their prevention.

4. The aims and methods in the food industry changed and the number of businesses linked to it increased significantly.

Surprisingly, the clinical qualification systems of different foods produced by international authorities (including Food and Drug Administration (FDA in the USA) differ from those in the case of drug production.

5. The consumption of different antibiotics (with and without medically based indications) increased in the last decades (see eradication treatment of the peptic ulcer patients), producing as side effects changes in the gut bacterial flora.

All of the abovementioned facts call our attention to the study of gut microbiome. At the moment, we are not able to confirm that changes in the gut microbiome are caused or are a consequence of the abovementioned processes; however, the link is strong.

The studies in this book give important information on the role of gut microbiome in the development of different diseases and their prevention. The chapters are written by researchers from the USA, China, Canada, and India. These chapters open new gates to understand the importance of gut microbiome. We have to be aware that these types of gut microbiome are an essential part of different research fields.

The editor is especially thankful on the excellent supports given by Ms. Ana Pantar (Senior Commissioning Editor) and by Ms. Romina Rovan (Publishing Process Manager) from InTech Open Access Publisher. Without their help, the publication of this book would not be possible.

Gyula Mozsik, MD, PhD, ScD
University of Pécs Medical School,
Hungary

Section 1

Non-Alcoholic Fatty Liver Disease, Gut Microbiota, Pro- and Prebiotics

Chapter 1

Nonalcoholic Fatty Liver Disease in Children: Role of the Gut Microbiota

Ding-You Li, Min Yang, Sitang Gong and
Shui Qing Ye

Additional information is available at the end of the chapter

http://dx.doi.org/10.5772/64799

Abstract

Nonalcoholic fatty liver disease (NAFLD) has emerged as the most common cause of liver disease among children and adolescents in industrialized countries due to increasing prevalence of obesity. It is generally recognized that both genetic and environmental risk factors contribute to the pathogenesis of NAFLD. Convincing evidences have shown that gut microbiota alteration is associated with NAFLD pathogenesis both in patients and animal models. Bacterial overgrowth and increased intestinal permeability are evident in NAFLD patients and lead to increased delivery of gut-derived bacterial products, such as lipopolysaccharide and bacterial DNA, to the liver through portal vein and then activation of toll-like receptors (TLRs), mainly TLR4 and TLR9, and their downstream cytokines and chemokines, resulting in hepatic inflammation. Currently, the role of gut microbiota in the pathogenesis of NAFLD is still the focus of many active clinical/basic researches. Modulation of gut microbiota with probiotics or prebiotics has been targeted as a preventive or therapeutic strategy on this pathological condition. Their beneficial effects on the NAFLD have been demonstrated in animal models and limited human studies.

Keywords: nonalcoholic fatty liver disease (NAFLD), children, gut microbiota, probiotics, prebiotics

1. Introduction

A growing obesity epidemic over the past three decades has become a major public health concern in developed as well as developing countries. According to the 2012 National Health and Nutrition Examination Survey [1, 2], in the United States, 35.5% of men, 35.8% of women,

INTECH
open science | open minds

© 2016 The Author(s). Licensee InTech. This chapter is distributed under the terms of the Creative Commons Attribution License (http://creativecommons.org/licenses/by/3.0), which permits unrestricted use, distribution, and reproduction in any medium, provided the original work is properly cited.

and 16.9% of children (2–19 years old) were considered obese. The worldwide prevalence of overweight and obesity increased from 28.8 to 36.9% in men, and from 29.8 to 38.0% in women between 1980 and 2013 [3]. Specifically, the prevalence for children increased from 16.9 to 23.8% for boys and from 16.2 to 22.6% for girls in developed countries, and from 8.1 to 12.9% for boys and from 8.4 to 13.4% for girls in developing countries as well [3].

Nonalcoholic fatty liver disease (NAFLD) has become the most common cause of liver disease in children in industrialized countries due to increasing prevalence of obesity [4]. NAFLD is defined as hepatic fat infiltration >5% of hepatocytes based on liver biopsy after excessive alcohol intake, viral, autoimmune, or drug-induced liver disease have been excluded. NAFLD is characterized by liver damage similar to that caused by alcohol but occurs in individuals that do not consume toxic quantities of alcohol. NAFLD includes a spectrum of liver diseases from simple fat infiltration (steatosis) through nonalcoholic steatohepatitis (NASH, steatosis with liver inflammation) to hepatic fibrosis and even hepatocellular carcinoma. The prevalence of NAFLD in the United States was 9.6% in normal weight children and 38% in obese ones based on liver biopsy at autopsy after accidents [5]. In the United States, the highest rates of pediatric NAFLD are in Hispanic and Asian children. In a study of 748 school children in Taiwan, the rates of NAFLD were 3% in the normal weight, 25% in the overweight, and 76% in the obese children determined by ultrasonography [6]. NAFLD in children is associated with severe obesity and metabolic syndrome, which includes abdominal obesity, type-2 diabetes, dyslipidemia, and hypertension. This chapter briefly summarizes the current understanding of the pathogenesis of NAFLD, role of gut microbiota, and potential new treatment strategies.

2. NAFLD pathogenesis: current understanding

Although the pathogenesis of NAFLD is not completely understood, considerable progresses have been made in recent years in explicating the mechanisms behind liver injury. As in other complex diseases, both genetic and environmental factors contribute to NAFLD development and progression. It is generally accepted that there is a genetic predisposition. In patients with NAFLD, genomic studies have identified many single nucleotide polymorphisms (SNPs) variants in genes controlling lipid metabolism, proinflammatory cytokines, fibrotic mediators, and oxidative stress. The most important one is the patatin-like phospholipase domain-containing 3 gene (PNPLA3) [7]. PNPLA3 rs738409 variant has been shown to confer susceptibility to NAFLD in obese children in different ethnic groups [8]. Other reported susceptible genes include glucokinase regulatory protein (GCKR), transmembrane 6 superfamily member 2 (TM6SF2), G-protein-coupled-receptor 120 (GPR120), farnesyl-diphosphate farnesyltransferase 1 (FDFT1), parvin beta (PARVB), sorting and assembly machinery component (SAMM50), lipid phosphate phosphatase-related protein type 4 (LPPR4), solute carrier family 38 member 8 (SLC38A8), lymphocyte cytosolic protein-1 (LCP1), group-specific component (GC), protein phosphatase 1 regulatory subunit 3b (PPP1R3B), lysophospholipase-like 1 (LYPLAL1), neurocan (NCAN), and polipoprotein C3 (APOC3) [9, 10]. To date, the strongest

SNP variants associated with pediatric NAFLD are the rs738409 in the *PNPLA3* gene, the 1260326 in the *GCKR* gene, and the rs58542926 in the *TM6SF2* gene.

Day and James initially proposed a two-hit hypothesis to explain the pathogenesis of NAFLD [11]. In individuals with genetic predisposition, the "first hit" results in liver fat accumulation (steatosis) due to environmental factors (e.g., western diet and lack of physical activity), obesity, insulin resistance, or metabolic syndrome. A subsequent "second hit", such as free fatty acids, adipokines/cytokines, oxidative stress (reactive oxygen species, lipid peroxidation), gut microbiota-derived endotoxins, mitochondrial dysfunction, and stellate cell activation, further amplify liver injury and NASH progression. A recent proposed multiple parallel hits hypothesis suggested that gut-derived and adipose tissue-derived factors may play a central role [12]. Both two-hit and multiple parallel hit hypotheses recognized that insulin resistance plays a crucial role in NAFLD pathogenesis and other factors including genetic determinants, nutritional factors, adipose tissue, and the immune system may be necessary for NAFLD manifestation and progression [11–13]. A new lipotoxicity hypothesis proposes that insulin resistance facilitates an excessive flow of free fatty acids to the liver, resulting in increased production of lipotoxic intermediates and eventually NASH, through oxidative stress, mitochondrial dysfunction, adiponectin, and other complex pathways [14, 15].

It has been well established that gut microbiota has been implicated in the development of NAFLD through the gut-liver axis [16–18]. An alteration of gut microbiota composition leads to bacterial overgrowth and increased intestinal permeability [19–21], resulting in translocation of gut micriobiota-derived products, such as lipopolysaccharide (LPS), bacterial DNA, and peptidoglycan, which would activate liver cell surface receptors (TLR4 and 9); a cascade of signal transductions is triggered and various cytokines and chemokines, such as TNF-α, TGF-β, IL-6, IL-10, CCL2, CCL5, and CxCL8, are released, leading to hepatic inflammation and fibrosis [22].

Evidences from both human and animal studies have supported important roles of gut microbiota-derived endotoxins, especially LPS, and their downstream signal pathways in the progression of NAFLD. Patients with NAFLD had increased serum endotoxin levels, with marked increases noted in NASH and early stage fibrosis. The increase in endotoxin level is related to IL-1α and TNF-α production [23–26]. In genetically obese fatty/fatty rats and obese/obese mice, Yang et al. showed that LPS contributes to the development of steatohepatitis by sensitizing TNF-α [27].

Toll-like receptors (TLRs) have been shown to play a crucial role in pathogenesis of NAFLD. Activation of TLRs and the adaptor molecule, MyD88, results in a cascade of signal transduction leading to release of various cytokines (TNF-α, TGF-β, interleukin-6 (IL-6), and IL-10) and chemokines (CCL2, CCL5, and CXCL8), which have been associated with NAFLD progression and hepatic fibrosis, as demonstrated in both human and animal studies [28]. TLRs are a class of pattern recognizing proteins that perceive bacterial and viral components. Gut microbiota is a source of TLR ligands, which can stimulate production of proinflammatory cytokines in the liver. TLRs are expressed on Kupffer cells, biliary epithelial cells, hepatocytes, hepatic stellate cells, epithelial cells, and dendritic cells in the liver. Among 13 known TLRs, TLR2, TLR4, and TLR9 have been implicated in NAFLD pathogenesis [17].

TLR4 is mainly activated by LPS, a cell component of Gram-negative bacteria. Elevated plasma and portal LPS levels are evident in human and animals with NAFLD [25, 29–32]. In methionine choline deficient diet(MCDD)-induced mouse model of NASH, liver injury and inflammatory cytokine production increased after challenge with LPS [33]. Rivera et al. further demonstrated histological change typical of steatohepatitis (extensive macrovesicular steatosis and necrosis), three-fold increase of portal blood endotoxin level, and enhanced TLR4 expression in wild-type mice fed with MCDD [31]. In a mouse model of high-fat diet-induced NAFLD, TLR4 signaling is involved in free fatty-acid-induced NF-kB activation in hepatocytes through release of free high-mobility group box1 (HMGB1), which is a key molecule for the activation of the TLR4/MyD88-dependent pathway [34]. TLR4 mutant mice fed with fructose-enriched diet had significantly less hepatic steatosis and lower TNFα levels in comparison to fructose-fed wild-type mice, indicating an important role of LPS/TLR4 signaling in fructose-induced NAFLD [35]. Plasma LPS levels are also markedly elevated in children and adults with NAFLD [25, 29, 30, 32]. Thus, gut microbiota-derived LPS/TLR4 signaling pathway is crucial for the progression of NAFLD in humans as well as animal models.

TLR9 is activated by bacterial DNA CpG motif and induces proinflammatory cytokine production. In a mouse model of CDAA diet-induced NASH, Miura et al. showed hepatic inflammation and fibrosis in wild-type mice, which was suppressed in mice deficient in TLR9 or MyD88, suggesting the critical role of the TLR9/MyD88 signaling pathway in the pathogenesis of NASH [36].

Inflammasomes have been shown to be major contributors to inflammation and are upregulated in mouse models of MCDD or high-fat-induced NASH and in livers of NASH patients. Stimulation of TLR4 by LPS can further activate inflammasomes [37]. In genetic inflammasome-deficiency mice, an altered gut microbiota configuration is associated with abnormal TLR4 and TLR9 agonist accumulation in the portal circulation, resulting in elevated hepatic TNF-α expression and exacerbation of hepatic steatosis and inflammation [38].

TLR2 recognizes components from Gram-positive and Gram-negative bacteria, as well as mycoplasma and yeast. In comparison to wild-type mice, TLR2-deficiency animals are substantially protected from high-fat diet-induced adiposity, insulin resistance, hypercholesterolemia, and hepatic steatosis [39]. In contrast, increased hepatic inflammation and TNF-α mRNA expression were observed in TLR2-deficiency mice fed with MCDD [33, 40]. The conflicting results of the role of TLR2 signaling in those studies could be due to different animal models used, different gut microbial ligands involved or compensation by other TLRs.

3. Modulation of gut microbiota: effects of prebiotics and probiotics on NAFLD

Given the accumulating evidence of the critical role of gut microbiota in the pathogenesis of NAFLD, microbiota manipulation has been targeted as a potentially therapeutic option for this pathological condition. Possible strategies for altering gut microbiota include probiotics, prebiotics, synbiotics, antibiotics, dietary modification/supplementation, and microbiota transplantation. So far, only probiotics have been tested for the treatment of NAFLD in animal models and human subjects with promising effects.

Probiotics are live commensal microorganisms that have been shown to beneficially modulate the host's gut microbiota. In animal models of NAFLD, VSL#3 (a probiotic mixture containing *streptococcus*, *Bifidobacterium*, and *lactobacillus*) improved hepatic inflammation and decreased hepatic steatosis with reduction of serum alanine aminotransferase (ALT) levels. Those changes were associated with decreased hepatic expression of TNF-mRNA and reduced activity of Jun N-terminal kinase (JNK) [41–43]. In methionine choline deficient diet (MCDD)-induced NASH rats treated with probiotic mixture containing 6 or 13 bacterial strains, which were isolated from the healthy human stool samples, improved hepatic inflammation, likely in part through modulation of TNF-α activity [44]. Furthermore, the treatment of apolipoprotein E-deficiency mice with dextran sulfate sodium (DSS) induced histopathological features typical of steatohepatitis, which were prevented by 12-week VSL#3 administration, through modulation of the expression of nuclear receptors, peroxisome proliferator-activated receptor-γ, Farnesoid-X-receptors, and vitamin D receptor [45].

In human studies, Aller et al. reported that a 3-month treatment with *Lactobacillus bulgaricus* and *Streptococcus thermophilus* improved liver aminotransferases in adult patients with NAFLD [46]. Alisi et al. performed a double-blind and placebo-controlled RCT to assess the effect of VSL#3 in 44 obese children with biopsy-proven NAFLD and demonstrated that VSL#3 supplement for 4 months significantly improved hepatic steatosis and BMI [47].

Prebiotics are nondigestible dietary fibers that stimulate the growth and activity of intestinal bacteria. In genetically obese mice, supplementation with prebiotics (oligofructose, a mix of fermentable dietary fibers) decreased plasma levels of LPS and cytokines (TNF-α, IL1b, IL1α, IL6, and INFγ) and reduced gut permeability through a mechanism involving glucagon-like peptide-2 [48]. Lactulose, as a prebiotic, can promote the growth of certain intestinal bacteria such as *Lactobacillus* and *Bifidobacterium*. In a rat model of high-fat diet-induced steatohepatitis, lactulose improved hepatic inflammatory activity and decreased serum endotoxin levels [49]. Human studies with prebiotics are very limited. In an earlier clinical pilot study in patients with biopsy-proven NASH, dietary supplementation of oligofructose 16 g/day for 8 weeks significantly decreased serum aminotransferases and insulin levels [50]. There have been no randomized, controlled, double-blind, prospective clinical trials of prebiotics on NAFLD, except a randomized controlled trial protocol, which will randomize adults with confirmed NAFLD to either a 16 g/day prebiotic supplemented group or isocaloric placebo group for 24 weeks (n = 30/group) [51].

4. NAFLD in children

4.1. Gut microbiota and NAFLD in children

Given the important role of gut microbiota in obesity and metabolic syndrome [52, 53], it is not surprising that ever-increasing literature in recent years suggested a potential role of gut microbiota in NAFLD pathogenesis. An observation by Spencer et al. provided the initial evidence that gut microbiota and human fatty liver are closely linked [54]. In adult subjects with choline-deficient diet-induced fatty liver, gut microbiota compositions were associated with changes in liver fat in each subject during choline depletion. Subsequently, Mouzaki et al. showed that patients with NASH had a lower percentage of Bacteroidetes compared to both simple steatosis and healthy controls and higher fecal *Clostridium coccoides* compared to those with simple steatosis [55]. There was an inverse and diet/BMI-independent association between the presence of NASH and percentage of Bacteroidetes, suggesting a link between gut microbiota and NAFLD severity. Raman et al. reported an over-representation of *Lactobacillus* species and selected members of phylum Firmicutes (Lachnospiraceae; genera, Dorea, Robinsoniella, and Roseburia) in NAFLD patients [56]. A recent study identified Bacteroides as independently associated with NASH and Ruminococcus with significant fibrosis and further confirmed the association of NAFLD severity with gut dysbiosis [57].

In a pediatric cohort of 63 children, Zhu et al. determined the composition of gut bacterial communities of obese children with NASH [58]. They found that Bacteroidetes were significantly elevated (mainly *Prevotella*) in obese and NASH patients compared to lean healthy children and that an increased abundance of ethanol-producing *Escherichia* in NASH children was observed. Ethanol can promote gut permeability. A recent study by Michail et al. showed that children with NAFLD had more abundant Gammaproteobacteria and Prevotella and significantly higher levels of ethanol, with differential effects on short chain fatty acids [59]. Both studies demonstrated that the gut microbiota profile in pediatric NAFLD is different from lean healthy children, with more ethanol-producing bacteria, suggesting that endogenous alcohol production by intestinal microbiota may play a role in NAFLD pathogenesis. Engstler et al. also showed that fasting ethanol levels were positively associated with measures of insulin resistance and significantly higher in children with NAFLD than in controls [60]. Interestingly, with further animal experiments, they demonstrated that increased blood ethanol levels in children with NAFLD may result from insulin-dependent impairments of alcohol dehydrogenase activity in liver tissue rather than from an increased endogenous ethanol synthesis [60]. Taken together, human studies demonstrated significant differences in gut microbiota between normal subjects and patients with NAFLD. However, there were great variations in microbiota compositions among these human studies, likely due to patient's age, fatty liver disease stages, study design, methods used, and observation endpoints.

4.2. Current management guidelines

All children with BMI ≥ 95th percentile or 85–94th percentile with risk factors (e.g., central obesity, metabolic syndrome, and strong family history) are recommended to have liver function test and hepatic ultrasonography [4, 61]. Since infants and children < 3 years old with fatty liver are less likely to have NAFLD, tests should be performed to exclude genetic, metabolic, syndromic, and systemic causes, such as fatty acid oxidation defects, lysosomal storage diseases, and peroxisomal disorders. In older children and teenagers, metabolic, infectious, toxic, and systemic causes should also be considered for differential diagnosis.

Recommended common laboratory tests include viral hepatitis panel, α-1 antitrypsin phenotype, ceruloplasmin, antinuclear antibody, lipid profile, TSH, and celiac panel.

Ultrasonography is the only imaging technique used for NAFLD screening in children because it is safe, noninvasive, widely available, relatively inexpensive, and can detect evidence of portal hypertension. Liver biopsy is recommended to exclude other treatable disease, in cases of clinically suspected advanced liver disease, before pharmacological/surgical treatment, and as part of a structured intervention protocol or clinical research trial [4, 61].

Treatment options for children with NAFLD are limited by a small number of randomized clinical trials and insufficient information on the natural history of the condition to assess risk-benefit ratios [4, 62]. So far, weight loss, though hard to achieve, is still the cornerstone of treatment regimen. Koot et al. demonstrated that a lifestyle intervention (physical exercise, dietary change, and behavioral modification) of 6 months significantly improved hepatic steatosis and serum aminotransferases in 144 children with NAFLD [63]. A long-term follow-up study showed that the greatest decrease of NAFLD prevalence was observed in children with the greatest overweight reduction [64]. Grønbæk et al. assessed the effect of a 10-week "weight loss camp" (restricted caloric intake and moderate exercise for one hour daily) in 117 obese children and found that the children had an average weight loss of 7.1 ± 2.7 kg, with significant improvements in hepatic steatosis, transaminases, and insulin sensitivity [65].

In children with poor adherence to lifestyle changes, pharmacological interventions and dietary supplementations, including antioxidants (vitamin E), insulin sensitizers (metoformin), ursodeoxycholic acid (UDCA), omega-3 docosahexaenoic acid (DHA), and probiotics, may be tried, but no randomized clinical trials have proved their effectiveness in children with NAFLD.

5. Summary and future directions

The increase of pediatric NAFLD is attributed to the worldwide obesity epidemic. Current evidences suggest that both genetic and environmental risk factors play a crucial role in the pathogenesis of NAFLD in children and adolescents. Although human studies clearly showed significant differences in gut microbiota between normal subjects and patients with NAFLD, there were great variations in microbiota compositions among these studies [66]. Adult patients have altered gut microbiota with an increase in the relative proportion of Bacteroidales and Clostridiales, whereas in children with NAFLD, ethanol-producing bacteria are predominant. Bacterial overgrowth and increased intestinal permeability are evident in NAFLD patients and lead to increased delivery of gut-derived bacterial products (e.g., LPS and bacterial DNA) to the liver through portal vein and then activation of toll-like receptors (TLRs), mainly TLR4 and TLR9, and their downstream cytokines and chemokines, resulting in hepatic inflammation [17].

Given the accumulating evidence of the critical role of gut-derived microbial factors in the development and/or progression of NAFLD, modulation of gut microbiota with probiotics and/or prebiotics has been targeted as a therapeutic option. Their beneficial effects on NALFD are promising based on studies in animal models and patients including children. However, before probiotics and prebiotics become prime-time therapeutic modalities for NAFLD in children, several issues need to be addressed. First, we still do not know whether all children with NAFLD are truly associated with altered intestinal microbiota, and if so, which microbiota is involved. Second, randomized clinical trials with appropriate powers are required to assess benefits of tailored interventions with probiotics and/or prebiotics in children with NAFLD. Finally, it is clinically important to know the best types of probiotics or prebiotics to be prescribed in children with NAFLD. Nevertheless, probiotics and other integrated strategies to modify intestinal microbiota are promising to become efficacious therapeutic modalities to treat NALFD, with emerging evidence to demonstrate that prebiotics and probiotics modulate the intestinal microbiota, improve epithelial barrier function, and reduce intestinal inflammation.

Author details

Ding-You Li[1*], Min Yang[2], Sitang Gong[2] and Shui Qing Ye[3]

*Address all correspondence to: dyli@cmh.edu

1 Department of Pediatrics, Children's Mercy Kansas City, University of Missouri School of Medicine, Kansas City, USA

2 Guangzhou Women and Children's Medical Center, Guangzhou Medical University, Guangzhou, China

3 Children's Mercy Kansas City, University of Missouri School of Medicine, Kansas City, USA

References

[1] Flegal KM, Carroll MD, Kit BK, Ogden CL: Prevalence of obesity and trends in the distribution of body mass index among US adults, 1999–2010. JAMA 2012; 307:491–497. DOI: 10.1001/jama.2012.39

[2] Ogden CL, Carroll MD, Kit BK, Flegal KM: Prevalence of obesity and trends in body mass index among US children and adolescents, 1999–2010. JAMA 2012; 307:483–490. DOI: 10.1001/jama.2012.40

[3] Ng M, Fleming T, Robinson M, et al: Global, regional, and national prevalence of overweight and obesity in children and adults during 1980–2013: a systematic analysis

for the Global Burden of Disease Study 2013. Lancet 2014; 384:766–781. DOI: 10.1016/S0140-6736(14)60460-8

[4] Vajro P, Lenta S, Socha P, Dhawan A, McKiernan P, Baumann U, Durmaz O, Lacaille F, McLin V, Nobili V: Diagnosis of nonalcoholic fatty liver disease in children and adolescents: position paper of the ESPGHAN Hepatology Committee. J Pediatr Gastroenterol Nutr. 2012; 54:700–713. DOI: 10.1097/MPG.0b013e318252a13f

[5] Schwimmer JB, Deutsch R, Kahen T, Lavine JE, Stanley C, Behling C: Prevalence of fatty liver in children and adolescents. Pediatrics 2006; 118:1388–1393.

[6] Huang SC, Yang YJ: Serum retinol-binding protein 4 is independently associated with pediatric NAFLD and fasting triglyceride level. J Pediatr Gastroenterol Nutr. 2013; 56: 145–150. DOI: 10.1097/MPG.0b013e3182722aee

[7] Romeo S, Kozlitina J, Xing C, Pertsemlidis A, Cox D, Pennacchio LA, Boerwinkle E, Cohen JC, Hobbs HH: Genetic variation in PNPLA3 confers susceptibility to nonalcoholic fatty liver disease. Nat Genet. 2008; 40:1461–1465. DOI: 10.1038/ng.257

[8] Lin YC, Chang PF, Chang MH, Ni YH: Genetic variants in GCKR and PNPLA3 confer susceptibility to nonalcoholic fatty liver disease in obese individuals. Am J Clin Nutr. 2014; 99:869–874. DOI: 10.3945/ajcn.113.079749

[9] Marzuillo P, Miraglia del Giudice E, Santoro N: Pediatric fatty liver disease: role of ethnicity and genetics. World J Gastroenterol. 2014; 20:7347–7355. DOI: 10.3748/wjg.v20.i23.7347

[10] Marzuillo P, Grandone A, Perrone L, Miraglia Del Giudice E: Understanding the pathophysiological mechanisms in the pediatric non-alcoholic fatty liver disease: the role of genetics. World J Hepatol. 2015; 7:1439–1443. DOI: 10.4254/wjh.v7.i11.1439

[11] Day CP, James OF: Steatohepatitis: a tale of two "hits"? Gastroenterology 1998; 114:842–845.

[12] Tilg H, Moschen AR: Evolution of inflammation in nonalcoholic fatty liver disease: the multiple parallel hits hypothesis. Hepatology 2010; 52:1836–1846. DOI: 10.1002/hep.24001

[13] Yang M, Gong S, Ye SQ, Lyman B, Geng L, Chen P, Li DY: Non-alcoholic fatty liver disease in children: focus on nutritional interventions. Nutrients 2014; 6:4691–4705. DOI: 10.3390/nu6114691

[14] Neuschwander-Tetri BA: Hepatic lipotoxicity and the pathogenesis of nonalcoholic steatohepatitis: the central role of nontriglyceride fatty acid metabolites. Hepatology 2010; 52:774–788. DOI: 10.1002/hep.23719

[15] Bechmann LP, Kocabayoglu P, Sowa JP, Sydor S, Best J, Schlattjan M, Beilfuss A, Schmitt J, Hannivoort RA, Kilicarslan A, Rust C, Berr F, Tschopp O, Gerken G, Friedman SL, Geier A, Canbay A: Free fatty acids repress small heterodimer partner (SHP) activation

and adiponectin counteracts bile acid-induced liver injury in superobese patients with nonalcoholic steatohepatitis. Hepatology 2013; 57:1394–1406. DOI: 10.1002/hep.26225

[16] Compare D, Coccoli P, Rocco A, Nardone OM, De Maria S, Cartenì M, Nardone G: Gut-liver axis: the impact of gut microbiota on non alcoholic fatty liver disease. Nutr Metab Cardiovasc Dis. 2012; 22:471–476. DOI: 10.1016/j.numecd.2012.02.007

[17] Miura K, Ohnishi H: Role of gut microbiota and Toll-like receptors in nonalcoholic fatty liver disease. World J Gastroenterol. 2014; 20:7381–7391. DOI: 10.3748/wjg.v20.i23.7381

[18] Kirpich IA, Marsano LS, McClain CJ: Gut-liver axis, nutrition, and non-alcoholic fatty liver disease. Clin Biochem. 2015; 48:923–930. DOI: 10.1016/j.clinbiochem.2015.06.023

[19] Wigg AJ, Roberts-Thomson IC, Dymock RB, McCarthy PJ, Grose RH, Cummins AG: The role of small intestinal bacterial overgrowth, intestinal permeability, endotoxaemia, and tumour necrosis factor alpha in the pathogenesis of non-alcoholic steatohepatitis. Gut 2001; 48:206–211.

[20] Sabaté JM, Jouët P, Harnois F, Mechler C, Msika S, Grossin M, Coffin B: High prevalence of small intestinal bacterial overgrowth in patients with morbid obesity: a contributor to severe hepatic steatosis. Obes Surg. 2008; 18:371–377. DOI: 10.1007/s11695-007-9398-2

[21] Miele L, Valenza V, La Torre G, Montalto M, Cammarota G, Ricci R, Mascianà R, Forgione A, Gabrieli ML, Perotti G, Vecchio FM, Rapaccini G, Gasbarrini G,Day CP, Grieco A: Increased intestinal permeability and tight junction alterations in nonalcoholic fatty liver disease. Hepatology 2009; 49:1877–1887. DOI: 10.1002/hep.22848

[22] Li DY, Yang M, Edwards S, Ye SQ: Non-alcoholic fatty liver disease: for better or worse, blame gut microbiota? JPEN J Parenter Enteral Nutr. 2013; 37:787–793. DOI: 10.1177/0148607113481623

[23] Poniachik J, Csendes A, Díaz JC, Rojas J, Burdiles P, Maluenda F, Smok G, Rodrigo R, Videla LA: Increased production of IL-1alpha and TNF-alpha in lipopolysaccharide-stimulated blood from obese patients with non-alcoholic fatty liver disease. Cytokine 2006; 33:252–257.

[24] Ruiz AG, Casafont F, Crespo J, Cayón A, Mayorga M, Estebanez A, Fernadez-Escalante JC, Pons-Romero F: Lipopolysaccharide-binding protein plasma levels and liver TNF-alpha gene expression in obese patients: evidence for the potential role of endotoxin in the pathogenesis of non-alcoholic steatohepatitis. Obes Surg. 2007; 17:1374–1380.

[25] Harte AL, da Silva NF, Creely SJ, McGee KC, Billyard T, Youssef-Elabd EM, Tripathi G, Ashour E, Abdalla MS, Sharada HM, Amin AI, Burt AD, Kumar S, Day CP, McTernan PG: Elevated endotoxin levels in non-alcoholic fatty liver disease. J Inflamm (Lond). 2010; 7:15. DOI: 10.1186/1476-9255-7-15

[26] Verdam FJ, Rensen SS, Driessen A, Greve JW, Buurman WA: Novel evidence for chronic exposure to endotoxin in human nonalcoholic steatohepatitis. J Clin Gastroenterol. 2011; 45:149–152. DOI: 10.1097/MCG.0b013e3181e12c24

[27] Yang SQ, Lin HZ, Lane MD, Clemens M, Diehl AM: Obesity increases sensitivity to endotoxin liver injury: implications for the pathogenesis of steatohepatitis. Proc Natl Acad Sci U S A. 1997; 94:2557–2562.

[28] Braunersreuther V, Viviani GL, Mach F, Montecucco F: Role of cytokines and chemokines in non-alcoholic fatty liver disease. World J Gastroenterol. 2012; 18:727–735.DOI: 10.3748/wjg.v18.i8.727

[29] Alisi A, Manco M, Devito R, Piemonte F, Nobili V: Endotoxin and plasminogen activator inhibitor-1 serum levels associated with nonalcoholic steatohepatitis in children. J Pediatr Gastroenterol Nutr. 2010; 50:645–649. DOI: 10.1097/MPG.0b013e3181c7bdf1

[30] Pendyala S, Walker JM, Holt PR: A high-fat diet is associated with endotoxemia that originates from the gut. Gastroenterology 2012; 142:1100–1101. DOI: 10.1053/j.gastro.2012.01.034

[31] Rivera CA, Adegboyega P, van Rooijen N, Tagalicud A, Allman M, Wallace M: Toll-like receptor-4 signaling and Kupffer cells play pivotal roles in the pathogenesis of non-alcoholic steatohepatitis. J Hepatol. 2007; 47:571–579.

[32] Sharifnia T, Antoun J, Verriere TG, Suarez G, Wattacheril J, Wilson KT, Peek RM Jr, Abumrad NN, Flynn CR: Hepatic TLR4 signaling in obese NAFLD. Am J Physiol Gastrointest Liver Physiol. 2015; 309:G270–278. DOI: 10.1152/ajpgi.00304.2014

[33] Szabo G, Velayudham A, Romics L Jr, Mandrekar P: Modulation of non-alcoholic steatohepatitis by pattern recognition receptors in mice: the role of toll-like receptors 2 and 4. Alcohol Clin Exp Res. 2005; 29(11Suppl):140S–145S.

[34] Li L, Chen L, Hu L, Liu Y, Sun HY, Tang J, Hou YJ, Chang YX, Tu QQ, Feng GS, Shen F, Wu MC, Wang HY: Nuclear factor high-mobility group box1 mediating the activation of Toll-like receptor 4 signaling in hepatocytes in the early stage of nonalcoholic fatty liver disease in mice. Hepatology 2011; 54:1620–1630. DOI: 10.1002/hep.24552

[35] Spruss A, Kanuri G, Wagnerberger S, Haub S, Bischoff SC, Bergheim I: Toll-like receptor 4 is involved in the development of fructose-induced hepatic steatosis in mice. Hepatology 2009; 50:1094–1104. DOI: 10.1002/hep.23122

[36] Miura K, Kodama Y, Inokuchi S, Schnabl B, Aoyama T, Ohnishi H, Olefsky JM, Brenner DA, Seki E: Toll-like receptor 9 promotes steatohepatitis by induction of interleukin-1beta in mice. Gastroenterology 2010; 139:323–334.e7. DOI: 10.1053/j.gastro.2010.03.052

[37] Csak T, Ganz M, Pespisa J, Kodys K, Dolganiuc A, Szabo G: Fatty acid and endotoxin activate inflammasomes in mouse hepatocytes that release danger signals to stimulate immune cells. Hepatology 2011; 54:133–144. DOI: 10.1002/hep.24341

[38] Henao-Mejia J, Elinav E, Jin C, Hao L, Mehal WZ, Strowig T, Thaiss CA, Kau AL, Eisenbarth SC, Jurczak MJ, Camporez JP, Shulman GI, Gordon JI, Hoffman HM, Flavell

RA: Inflammasome-mediated dysbiosis regulates progression of NAFLD and obesity. Nature 2012; 482:179–185. DOI: 10.1038/nature10809

[39] Himes RW, Smith CW: Tlr2 is critical for diet-induced metabolic syndrome in a murine model. FASEB J. 2010; 24:731–739. DOI: 10.1096/fj.09-141929

[40] Rivera CA, Gaskin L, Allman M, Pang J, Brady K, Adegboyega P, Pruitt K: Toll-like receptor-2 deficiency enhances non-alcoholic steatohepatitis. BMC Gastroenterol. 2010; 10:52. DOI: 10.1186/1471-230X-10-52

[41] Li Z, Yang S, Lin H, Huang J, Watkins PA, Moser AB, Desimone C, Song XY, Diehl AM: Probiotics and antibodies to TNF inhibit inflammatory activity and improve nonalcoholic fatty liver disease. Hepatology 2003; 37:343–350.

[42] Velayudham A, Dolganiuc A, Ellis M, Petrasek J, Kodys K, Mandrekar P, Szabo G: VSL#3 probiotic treatment attenuates fibrosis without changes in steatohepatitis in a diet-induced nonalcoholic steatohepatitis model in mice. Hepatology 2009; 49:989–997. DOI: 10.1002/hep.22711

[43] Xu RY, Wan YP, Fang QY, Lu W, Cai W: Supplementation with probiotics modifies gut flora and attenuates liver fat accumulation in rat nonalcoholic fatty liver disease model. J. Clin Biochem Nutr. 2012; 50:72–77. DOI: 10.3164/jcbn.11-38

[44] Karahan N, Işler M, Koyu A, Karahan AG, Başyığıt Kiliç G, Cırış IM, Sütçü R, Onaran I, Cam H, Keskın M: Effects of probiotics on methionine choline deficient diet-induced steatohepatitis in rats. Turk J Gastroenterol. 2012; 23:110–121.

[45] Mencarelli A, Cipriani S, Renga B, Bruno A, D'Amore C, Distrutti E, Fiorucci S: VSL#3 resets insulin signaling and protects against NASH and atherosclerosis in a model of genetic dyslipidemia and intestinal inflammation. PLoS One 2012; 7:e45425. DOI: 10.1371/journal.pone.0045425

[46] Aller R, De Luis DA, Izaola O, Conde R, Gonzalez Sagrado M, Primo D, De La Fuente B, Gonzalez J: Effect of a probiotic on liver aminotransferases in nonalcoholic fatty liver disease patients: a double blind randomized clinical trial. Eur Rev Med Pharmacol Sci. 2011; 15:1090–1095.

[47] Alisi A, Bedogni G, Baviera G, Giorgio V, Porro E, Paris C, Giammaria P, Reali L, Anania F, Nobili V: Randomised clinical trial: the beneficial effects of VSL#3 in obese children with non-alcoholic steatohepatitis. Aliment Pharmacol Ther 2014; 39:1276–1285. DOI: 10.1111/apt.12758

[48] Cani PD, Possemiers S, Van de Wiele T, Guiot Y, Everard A, Rottier O, Geurts L, Naslain D, Neyrinck A, Lambert DM, Muccioli GG, Delzenne NM: Changes in gut microbiota control inflammation in obese mice through a mechanism involving GLP-2-driven improvement of gut permeability. Gut 2009; 58:1091–1103. DOI: 10.1136/gut.2008.165886

[49] Fan JG, Xu ZJ, Wang GL: Effect of lactulose on establishment of a rat non-alcoholic steatohepatitis model. World J Gastroenterol. 2005; 11:5053–5056.

[50] Daubioul CA, Horsmans Y, Lambert P, Danse E, Delzenne NM: Effects of oligofructose on glucose and lipid metabolism in patients with nonalcoholic steatohepatitis: results of a pilot study. Eur J Clin Nutr. 2005; 59:723–726.

[51] Lambert JE, Parnell JA, Eksteen B, Raman M, Bomhof MR, Rioux KP, Madsen KL, Reimer RA: Gut microbiota manipulation with prebiotics in patients with non-alcoholic fatty liver disease: a randomized controlled trial protocol. BMC Gastroenterol. 2015; 15:169. DOI: 10.1186/s12876-015-0400-5

[52] Turnbaugh PJ, Ley RE, Mahowald MA, Magrini V, Mardis ER, Gordon JI: An obesity-associated gut microbiome with increased capacity for energy harvest. Nature. 2006; 444:1027–1031.

[53] Nicholson JK, Holmes E, Kinross J, Burcelin R, Gibson G, Jia W, Pettersson S: Host-gut microbiota metabolic interactions. Science 2012; 336:1262–1267. DOI: 10.1126/science.1223813

[54] Spencer MD, Hamp TJ, Reid RW, Fischer LM, Zeisel SH, Fodor AA: Association between composition of the human gastrointestinal microbiome and development of fatty liver with choline deficiency. Gastroenterology 2011; 140:976–986. DOI: 10.1053/j.gastro.2010.11.049

[55] Mouzaki M, Comelli EM, Arendt BM, Bonengel J, Fung SK, Fischer SE, McGilvray ID, Allard JP: Intestinal microbiota in patients with nonalcoholic fatty liver disease. Hepatology 2013; 58:120–127. DOI: 10.1002/hep.26319

[56] Raman M, Ahmed I, Gillevet PM, Probert CS, Ratcliffe NM, Smith S, Greenwood R, Sikaroodi M, Lam V, Crotty P, Bailey J, Myers RP, Rioux KP: Fecal microbiome and volatile organic compound metabolome in obese humans with nonalcoholic fatty liver disease. Clin Gastroenterol Hepatol. 2013; 11:868–875. e1-3. DOI: 10.1016/j.cgh.2013.02.015

[57] Boursier J, Mueller O, Barret M, Machado M, Fizanne L, Araujo-Perez F, Guy CD, Seed PC, Rawls JF, David LA, Hunault G, Oberti F, Calès P, Diehl AM: The severity of NAFLD is associated with gut dysbiosis and shift in the metabolic function of the gut microbiota. Hepatology 2016; 63:764–775. DOI: 10.1002/hep.28356

[58] Zhu L, Baker SS, Gill C, Liu W, Alkhouri R, Baker RD, Gill SR: Characterization of gut microbiomes in nonalcoholic steatohepatitis (NASH) patients: a connection between endogenous alcohol and NASH. Hepatology 2013; 57:601–609. DOI: 10.1002/hep.26093

[59] Michail S, Lin M, Frey MR, Fanter R, Paliy O, Hilbush B, Reo NV: Altered gut microbial energy and metabolism in children with non-alcoholic fatty liver disease. FEMS Microbiol Ecol. 2015; 91:1–9. DOI: 10.1093/femsec/fiu002

[60] Engstler AJ, Aumiller T, Degen C, Dürr M, Weiss E, Maier IB, Schattenberg JM, Jin CJ, Sellmann C, Bergheim I: Insulin resistance alters hepatic ethanol metabolism: studies

in mice and children with non-alcoholic fatty liver disease. Gut. 2015. DOI: 10.1136/gutjnl-2014-308379. [Epub ahead of print]

[61] Nobili V, Alkhouri N, Alisi A, Della Corte C, Fitzpatrick E, Raponi M, Dhawan A: Nonalcoholic fatty liver disease: a challenge for pediatricians. JAMA Pediatr. 2015;169:170–176. DOI: 10.1001/jamapediatrics.2014.2702

[62] Chalasani N, Younossi Z, Lavine JE, Diehl AM, Brunt EM, Cusi K, Charlton M, Sanyal AJ: The diagnosis and management of non-alcoholic fatty liver disease: practice guideline by the American Association for the Study of Liver Diseases, American College of Gastroenterology, and the American Gastroenterological Association. Hepatology 2012; 55:2005–2023. DOI: 10.1002/hep.25762

[63] Koot BG, van der Baan-Slootweg OH, Tamminga-Smeulders CL, Rijcken TH, Korevaar JC, van Aalderen WM, Jansen PL, Benninga MA: Lifestyle intervention for non-alcoholic fatty liver disease: prospective cohort study of its efficacy and factors related to improvement. Arch Dis Child. 2011; 96:669–674. DOI: 10.1136/adc.2010.199760

[64] Reinehr T, Schmidt C, Toschke AM, Andler W: Lifestyle intervention in obese children with non-alcoholic fatty liver disease: 2-year follow-up study. Arch Dis Child. 2009; 94:437–442. DOI: 10.1136/adc.2008

[65] Grønbæk H, Lange A, Birkebæk NH, Holland-Fischer P, Solvig J, Hørlyck A, Kristensen K, Rittig S, Vilstrup H: Effect of a 10-week weight loss camp on fatty liver disease and insulin sensitivity in obese Danish children. J Pediatr Gastroenterol Nutr. 2012; 54:223–228. DOI: 10.1097/MPG.0b013e31822cdedf

[66] Wieland A, Frank DN, Harnke B, Bambha K: Systematic review: microbial dysbiosis and nonalcoholic fatty liver disease. Aliment Pharmacol Ther. 2015; 42:1051–1063. DOI: 10.1111/apt.13376

Section 2

Human Gastrointestinal Tract Diseases and Gut Dysbacteriosis

Chapter 2

The Pathology of Methanogenic Archaea in Human Gastrointestinal Tract Disease

Suzanne L. Ishaq, Peter L. Moses and
André-Denis G. Wright

Additional information is available at the end of the chapter

http://dx.doi.org/10.5772/64637

Abstract

Methane-producing archaea have recently been associated with disorders of the gastrointestinal tract and dysbiosis of the resident microbiota. Some of these conditions include inflammatory bowel disease (Crohn's disease (CD) and ulcerative colitis (UC)), chronic constipation, small intestinal bacterial overgrowth, gastrointestinal cancer, anorexia, and obesity. The causal relationship and the putative mechanism by which archaea may be associated with human disease are poorly understood, as are the strategies to alter methanogen populations in humans. It is estimated that 30–62% of humans produce methane detectable in exhaled breath and in the gastrointestinal tract. However, it is not yet known what portion of the human population have detectable methanogenic archaea. Hydrogen and methane are often measured in the breath as clinical indicators of intolerance to lactose and other carbohydrates. Breath gas analysis is also employed to diagnose suspected small intestinal bacterial overgrowth and irritable bowel syndrome, although standards are lacking. The diagnostic value for breath gas measurement in human disease is evolving; therefore, standardized breath gas measurements combined with ever-improving molecular methodologies could provide novel strategies to prevent, diagnose, or manage numerous colonic disorders. In cases where methanogens are potentially pathogenic, more data are required to develop therapeutic antimicrobials or other mitigation strategies.

Keywords: methanogens, colorectal cancer, irritable bowel syndrome, methane

INTECH
open science | open minds

© 2016 The Author(s). Licensee InTech. This chapter is distributed under the terms of the Creative Commons Attribution License (http://creativecommons.org/licenses/by/3.0), which permits unrestricted use, distribution, and reproduction in any medium, provided the original work is properly cited.

1. Introduction

1.1. Methanogen diversity in the gastrointestinal tract

Archaea represent the third domain of life, in addition to Prokaryota, which they more or less physically resemble, and Eukaryota, with which they have more genetic similarities. Many archaea are classified as extremophiles, but those which live in the digestive tract of animals are known as methanogens. Archaeal diversity in the gastrointestinal tract (GIT) is far less than that of bacteria, and more specifically monogastrics have a much lower diversity as compared to herbivorous ruminant animals. In both host types, species belonging to the genus *Methanobrevibacter* have been cited as the dominant methanogens in the GIT. In fact, *Mbr. smithii* is the dominant species found in the human GIT, followed by *Methanosphaera stadtmanae* [1–5]. This lack of relative diversity is largely a function of diet, the presence or absence of other microorganisms, or digestive tract physiology, but it may play a role in human intestinal dysbiosis. A general increase in microbial diversity has been correlated with a healthy gut microbiome that is resistant to physical or biotic disruptions, as there is redundancy in metabolic pathways and the increased competition precludes dominance by one particular taxon. Higher methanogen diversity was correlated with lower breath methane production in humans [1].

Methanogens use hydrogen, in the form of free protons, H_2 gas, NADH and NADPH cofactors, acetate, or formate, to reduce carbon dioxide and produce methane gas. Thus, methanogens rely on the by-products of bacterial fermentation of carbohydrates (i.e., carbon, hydrogen, acetate, formate, or methanol) as precursor materials required for methanogenesis and their own energy production. Dietary carbohydrates which are not broken down or absorbed by the host are available to bacteria for fermentation [6], and a large amount of unused carbohydrates may consequently increase bacterial fermentation and archaeal methanogenesis. A diet high in fiber and structural carbohydrates, which are largely indigestible to animal and human enzymes (i.e., cellulose, hemicellulose, and lignin), is associated with populations of *Methanobrevibacter ruminantium* [7], while a diet high in starch and other easily digestible carbohydrates is associated with *Mbr. smithii* [8, 9]. *Mbr. smithii* has been shown to improve polysaccharide digestion by GIT bacteria and fungi, and even influence the production of acetate or formate for its own use [10, 11]. *Msp. stadtmanae* requires methanol, a compound that is the by-product of pectin fermentation, for its methanogenesis pathway, which accounts for its presence in omnivores [1, 2, 5, 12].

Methanogens also have a slower growth rate than bacteria, which is sensitive to concentrations of hydrogen required as an electron donor during methanogenesis, as well as other nutrients. Few methanogenic taxa are motile, and these are limited to the order Methanococcales, and the genera *Methanospirillum, Methanolobus, Methanogenium*, and *Methanomicrobium* (order: Methanomicrobiales) [13, 14]. This difficulty of remaining situated in the intestines is a limiting factor in methanogen density. In humans, methanogens tend to be denser in the left colon, where fecal matter becomes more solid and transit time slows down [15], but they have also been found in the small intestine [16]. In addition, passing through the gastric stomach is challenging, which may explain why oral and intestinal populations of archaea and bacteria do not share an overlapping diversity [17, 18]. To overcome challenges to intestinal retention, some species of methanogens have adapted to the human colon and are able to thrive. *Mbr. smithii* produces surface glycans and adhesion-like proteins which improves their interaction with host epithelia and allows for persistence in the gut, as well as wider range of fermentation by-products, which can be used for methanogenesis, allowing for the flexibility of the human diet [3].

1.2. Intestinal methane and the effect on the host

Colonic gases are among the most tangible features of digestion, yet physicians are typically unable to offer long-term relief from clinical complaints related to excessive gas and associated discomfort. Studies characterizing colonic gases have linked changes in volume or composition to individuals with gastrointestinal disorders (see below). These studies have suggested that hydrogen gas, methane, hydrogen sulfide, and carbon dioxide are by-products related to the interplay between hydrogen-producing fermentative bacteria and hydrogen consumers (reductive acetogenic bacteria, sulfate-reducing bacteria, and methanogenic archaea). The primary benefit of methanogenesis in the GIT is to decrease hydrogen (hydrogen gas, NADH, NADPH) resulting from carbohydrate fermentation by bacteria, protozoa, and fungi [19]. Hydrogen gas in the intestines can shorten intestinal transit times of feces by 10–47% [20]. Moreover, hydrogen has been shown to have antioxidant properties as an oxygen scavenger [21, 22]. It is possible that in the healthy colon, physiological hydrogen concentrations might protect the mucosa from oxidative insults, whereas an impaired hydrogen economy might facilitate inflammation or carcinogenesis.

However, excessive hydrogen in the GIT can be detrimental to commensal microorganisms. The decrease in hydrogen through the generation of inert methane gas helps to prevent hydrogen damage to host or symbiotic microbial cells [23]. In ruminant animals, which have a four-chambered stomach, methanogens associated with ciliate protozoa act as a hydrogen sink [24], especially in the first two stomach chambers, the rumen and reticulum. There are a few commensal protozoan species that can be found in the human intestinal tract [25], but it is not yet known if they symbiotically interact with methanogens. Generally, this interaction only occurs with protozoa that have a hydrogenosome organelle, which metabolizes pyruvate and uses hydrogen ions as electron acceptors. In humans, the only protozoa that have a hydrogenosome are trichomonads, such as *Trichomonas hominis* and *Trichomonas tenax*, both of which are nonpathogenic [25, 26].

Alternative hydrogen sinks in humans include sulfate-reducing bacteria (SRB), which produce hydrogen sulfide gas that is absorbed and detoxified by the liver, or acetogenic bacteria, which produce the short-chain fatty acid acetate that can be metabolized by the host or other microorganisms. Some of these pathways are mutually exclusive in humans, and either SRB or methanogens will be present in large numbers [27]. Although higher hydrogen sulfide and SRB levels have been detected in patients with irritable bowel disease (IBD), and to a lesser extent in colorectal cancer (CRC), this colonic gas might have beneficial effects as a gaso-transmitter [28]. Acetogens, on the other hand, have up to a 100 times higher hydrogen concentration threshold, and thus cannot out-compete methanogens for precursors [29, 30].

Consequently, acetogenesis is rare in the human GIT, and if present is usually restricted to the right colon [31].

Unlike hydrogen, there are as yet no known biological sinks for methane in the intestines [32], although methanotrophic bacteria exist in a variety of water and soil environments. Instead, some methane is excreted from the colon, and most is absorbed into the blood stream and expelled from the lungs via exhalation. This allows methane production to be indirectly and noninvasively measured, since breath methane concentration is correlated with methanogen cell density in the intestines [1]. An undetectable concentration of breath methane does not equate to the absence of archaea, and therefore false-negative interpretations of breath gas analysis may result when breath methane is at undetectably low levels [33, 34]. Reported estimations suggest that between 30 and 62% of healthy humans produce detectable methane [31, 35]. The presence of methane gas in the intestines may influence or reduce intestinal transit time, and the correlation between breath methane production and transit time has been observed even in healthy individuals [19]. This was further examined using animal models, in which the overabundance of methane gas caused a reduction in transit time while increasing intestinal contractions [20, 36], thus increasing pressure inside the intestine by an average of 137% [20]. Alteration of intestinal motility may benefit slow-growing methanogen populations, which are limited by their ability to attach to host mucosal epithelia and maintain themselves in the intestines.

This increased gas production and resulting pressure cause bloating, discomfort, flatulence, or belching. In addition to detrimental physical effects, it has been speculated that methane potentially causes chemical and biological effects as a "gaso-transmitter" [37], in the same way that hydrogen sulfide affects smooth muscle activity [37] or nitrous oxide (N_2O) is used in biological systems to control vascular tone [38]. Studies using isolated gastrointestinal tissue suggest that this interaction is between methane and enteric nervous tissue, rather than the central nervous system [20]. Clinically, hydrogen and methane measured in breath can indicate lactose and glucose intolerance, small-intestine bacterial overgrowth (SIBO), irritable bowel syndrome (IBS), or other gastrointestinal diseases [35, 36, 39–42]. Therefore, standardized breath gas measurements combined with ever-improving molecular methodologies could provide novel strategies to prevent, diagnose, or manage numerous colonic disorders as defined by the Rome III diagnostic criteria [43].

2. The role of archaea in metabolic disorders

Obesity in adults is most commonly defined using body mass index (BMI) (kg body weight/height in meters squared), and for Caucasian adults, is defined as a BMI of ≥30 kg/m^2. For over a decade, shifts in intestinal bacteria diversity have been associated with weight gain or obesity in humans, generally following an increase in the proportion of Firmicutes [44], a decrease in Bacteroidetes, which has shown some anti-obesity influences [44–46], and with a shift in more minor phyla. Generally, this shift in intestinal bacteria leads to an increase in host energy harvest by improving polysaccharide digestion and host epithelial absorption which, in turn, causes weight gain [47–49]. Alternatively, a change in host genetics or immune system function can also cause a shift in bacterial diversity. The lack of host immune-modulating factors, such as Toll-like receptor 5 (TLR5) and fasting-induced adipocyte factor (Fiaf), produced insulin resistance, increased adiposity (especially visceral), and shifted GIT bacterial diversity and functionality in mice [49, 50]. Additionally, endotoxinemia, or the presence of microbial endotoxins (e.g., lipopolysaccharide-A (LPS)) in intestines or blood, has been shown to induce obesity, glucose intolerance, weight gain, and adiposity in response to a high-fat diet [51–53].

It would seem that bacterial diversity and density may have a specific role in metabolic dysbiosis, as treatment with oral antibiotics has been shown effective at improving fasting and oral glucose tolerance test (OGTT) levels in obese or insulin-resistant mice [54], or mitigating endotoxinemia and reducing cecal LPS concentrations in mice on a high-fat diet [51, 55]. Both obesity and diabetes are also correlated with low-grade chronic intestinal inflammation, likely caused by bacterial LPS. The presence of LPS, among other systemic immune responses, causes host macrophages to express pro-inflammatory cytokines, and in adipose-associated macrophages this only increases local insulin resistance and lipid storage [51, 53].

More recent studies have focused on the shifts in archaea associated with high-fat/high-calorie diets or weight gain, especially as *Mbr. smithii* has been shown to increase polysaccharide digestion by bacteria and fungi [10, 11] and may play a specific role in increasing energy harvest. *Mbr. smithii* has been shown to increase in density in rats when switching to a high-fat diet, and was associated with higher weight gain when given as a supplement regardless of the diet [16]. In humans, BMI was higher in breath methane-positive subjects (45.2 ± 2.3 kg/m^2) than in breath methane-negative subjects (38.5 ± 0.8 kg/m^2, $P = 0.001$) [56]. In a separate study, methane- and hydrogen-positive subjects again had higher BMI than other groups (M+/H+ 26.5 ± 7.1 kg/m^2, $P < 0.02$), and also had significantly higher percent body fat (M+/H+ $34.1 \pm 10.9\%$, $P < 0.001$) [41]. Interestingly, *Mbr. smithii* density was found to be highly elevated in anorexic patients (5.26×10^8 rRNA copies/g feces), even more so than in obese patients (1.68×10^8 rRNA copies/g feces), as compared to healthy bodyweight subjects (9.78×10^7 rRNA copies/g feces) [57].

Obesity is strongly associated with an increased risk for diabetes mellitus, or type-2 diabetes, which is an inducible metabolic disease characterized by a lack of pancreatic production of insulin, or a resistance to insulin at the cellular level. Type-1 diabetes is an autoimmune disease characterized by the destruction of pancreatic beta cells which normally produce insulin. Diabetes can lead to a host of other health problems, most especially cardiovascular disease, renal failure, increased glaucoma and potential blindness, and reduced circulation, which increases the risk for ulcers and infection in the peripheral limbs. Few studies investigate the potential link between methanogens and diabetes. Type-1 diabetic patients with no complications showed a significant increase in intestinal transit time, although it was not associated with other gastric symptoms [58]. Type-1 diabetes with an autonomic diabetic neuropathy complication affects heart rate, blood pressure, perspiration, or digestion. Some patients with this neuropathy have also been positive for SIBO [59, 60], which was associated with an increased daily insulin requirement [60], or detectable methane production, which was associated with a worse glycemic index [59]. Breath methane producers, which had comparable BMI and baseline insulin resistance to non-methane producers, had higher serum glucose levels and a longer return to normal resting glucose after OGTT [61]. The mechanistic relationship between methanogens, methane, and diabetes has yet to be explained.

3. The role of archaea in colon cancer

Colorectal cancer is the most commonly diagnosed malignancy in the Western World, being the fourth most common cancer diagnosis in the United States but the second leading cause of cancer-related deaths [62]. In nonsmokers, it is the leading cause of cancer-related death in men and the second leading cause of cancer-related death in women (after breast cancer). The 5-year survival rate varies by stage and type, ranging from 53 to 92% [62]. All colorectal cancers originate from adenomas or flat dysplasia, and are often asymptomatic, though occult bleeding may result and ultimately may be associated with an unexplained iron deficiency anemia. Large tumors in the distal or left colon may result in a compromised bowel lumen and potentially lead to symptoms including constipation, diarrhea, or bowel obstruction. The histopathology of CRC is complicated and involves a number of differently defined molecular pathways. There is evidence of microbial dysbiosis in CRC patients, as well as higher levels of breath methane in patients with CRC and premalignant polyps, as presented below.

Viral causative agents have been identified in a variety of cancers, but it is only recently that prokaryotic- or eukaryotic-causative or protective agents have been investigated. Cancer has been associated with a reduced bacterial diversity in the digestive tract [63], as well as in the mammary glands [64]. Specific agents have been identified, which cause localized cancers through their molecular interactions with host cells [65], such as *Helicobacter pylori* in stomach cancers or a link between the diplomonad protozoan *Giardia* in pancreatic and gallbladder cancer, but no archaea have yet been cited as a possible agent [66]. A recent review by Gill and Brinkman [67] discusses the role of bacterial phages (viruses that exclusively infect bacteria) in bringing mobility and virulence factors to bacteria, while archaea are infected by archaeon-specific phages which are unlikely to have independently evolved similar virulence factors to bacterial phages. Additionally, while archaea and bacteria are both prokaryotic, though in different phylogenetic domains, there is little evidence of horizontal gene transfer between them [67].

There is some discussion about the change in the density of methanogens in individuals with colorectal cancer [33, 68, 69]. Methanogen density was shown to be inversely related to the fecal concentration of butyrate, a short-chain fatty acid produced by bacterial fermentation [70]. Butyrate has been shown to provide energy for digestive tract epithelia cells, upregulate host immune system and mucin production, alter toxic or mutagenic compounds, and reduce the size and number of crypt foci, which are abnormal glands in intestinal epithelia that lead to colorectal polyps [71–73]. An altered gut microbiome in colorectal patients could shift bacterial fermentation away from butyrate production to something more favorable to methanogenesis.

Methane production was increased in patients with precancerous symptoms and colorectal cancer [39, 74], and was directly proportional to constipation but inversely proportional to diarrhea in chemotherapy patients [75]. In the same study, pH was also directly proportional to constipation but inversely proportional to diarrhea in chemotherapy patients [75]. Methane itself has not been shown to be carcinogenic. However, the oxidation of methane forms formaldehyde, which is carcinogenic [76]. On the other hand, hydrogen sulfide gas produced by SRB has shown to promote angiogenesis (which tumors rely on), and has been shown to be genotoxic when DNA repair is inhibited [77]. Colon cancer biopsies have shown an increase in the enzyme cystathionine-β-synthase (CBS), which allows host cancer cells to produce their own hydrogen sulfide, and a silencing of this gene was able to reduce tumor cell growth, proliferation, and migration [78].

4. The role of archaea in irritable bowel syndrome

The symptoms of IBS vary between patients, and may include diarrhea, constipation, excess flatus secondary to hydrogen or methane production, bloating, abdominal pain, and visceral hypersensitivity [79]. Hydrogen sulfide gas from SRB was shown to increase luminal hypersensitivity [80]. In addition, IBS is associated with changes in the diversity and density of intestinal bacteria [42, 81–83], as well as with an increase in hydrogen production [84]. In some patients with IBS, the change in bacterial populations is amplified, leading to SIBO. SIBO is also seen in non-IBS patients, but it is much more prevalent in IBS patients, especially those with constipation as opposed to diarrhea [85, 86]. A common technique for the management of symptoms includes switching patients to a diet low in fermentable oligosaccharides, disaccharides, monosaccharides, and polyols (FODMAPs) [87]. Two-thirds of patients report symptoms linked to diet [88], especially gas production and bloating following ingestion of lactose [89], other carbohydrates, or fats [40, 88].

While the specific cause of IBS still remains unclear, the altered bacterial diversity causes a shift in carbohydrate fermentation and altered gas production. If this shift favors methanogenesis, the result is a decrease in transit time and an increase in constipation. The presence of methanogens in the digestive tract, and the production of methane, has been associated with patients with IBS, and especially with chronic constipation and reduced passage rate in the intestines (slow transit) [42, 85, 90]. Methanogen density was found to be lower in IBS patients as compared to controls [69, 91], although density and methane production were increased in IBS patients with constipation as compared to IBS patients without constipation [90]. *Methanobrevibacter* spp. are increased with diets high in easily digestible carbohydrates, but decreased in diets high in amino acids/proteins and fatty acids [8], specifically *Mbr. smithii* [9]. More specifically, *Mbr. smithii* was higher in IBS patients with constipation and higher methane production [90], and they have previously been shown as the dominant species in healthy individuals who have high methane production [1].

5. The role of archaea in inflammatory bowel disease

Contrary to recent findings in patients with IBS, low methane production [35, 42] and lower methanogen density [69] were seen in patients with IBD, which includes the specific entities Crohn's and ulcerative colitis. In contrast to IBS, IBD patients demonstrate chronic inflammatory changes in the colon (UC) or in the small bowel, or a combination of small bowel and colon involvement (CD).

Recently, it was demonstrated that two archaeal species normally found in the digestive system, *Mbr. smithii* and *Msp. stadtmanae*, can have differential immunogenic properties in the lungs of mice when aerosolized and inhaled [92]. Furthermore, *Msp. stadtmanae* was found to be a strong inducer of the inflammatory response [92], and it is likely that this may occur even in the GIT where it is normally found. Blais Lecours et al. [93] investigated the immunogenic potential of archaea in humans relating to patients with IBD. Mononuclear cells stimulated with *Msp. stadtmanae* produced higher concentrations of tumor necrosis factor (TNF) (39.5 ng/ml) compared to *Mbr. smithii* stimulation (9.1 ng/ml) [93]. Bacterial concentrations and frequency of *Mbr. smithii*-containing stools were similar in both healthy controls and patients with IBD; however, the number of stool samples positive for the inflammatory archaea *Msp. stadtmanae* was higher in patients than in controls (47 vs 20%) [93]. Importantly, only IBD patients developed a significant anti-*Msp. stadtmanae* immunoglobulin G (IgG) response [93], indicating that the composition of the microbiome appears to be an important determinate of the presence or absence of autoimmunity. Recent advances in mucosal immunology and culture-independent sequencing of the microbiome support the hypothesis that alterations in the microbiota can alter the host immune response as is observed in IBD [94]. A specific role for archaeal species has yet to be clearly defined.

6. The role of archaea in other intestinal dysbiosis

There are many rare gastrointestinal diseases and general conditions of dysbiosis which are not well understood, but which may have a link to methane production in the intestines. Pneumatosis cystoides intestinalis (PCI) is a condition in which gas-filled cysts occur in the smooth muscle wall of the intestines, where it cannot be relieved by flatulence. It is believed to be caused by bacteria in the intestinal wall. Interestingly, patients with PCI have lower prevalence of breath methane production than patients with IBS, CD, UC, and even healthy control subjects [35].

Non-IBS constipated patients with slow transit were more likely to have detectable levels of breath methane (75 vs 44%) than constipated patients with normal transit, and both were more likely to have detectable breath methane than nonconstipated controls (28%) [95]. This trend was also reported in other studies [56, 85].

Diverticulitis, a condition involving the herniation of the intestinal mucosal and submucosal layers back through the intestinal smooth muscle and creates pockets that harbor infections, has only been noted since the early 1800s [96]. Interestingly, it is most common in the left colon in subjects from Western countries and the right colon in subjects from Asian countries [96], which is likely a function of the "Western diet." Diverticulitis was associated with a high prevalence of methanogens in stool and high methane output [33], as well as fiber intake, age-associated changes in the colon wall, low colonic motility, and high intraluminal pressure; however, methane output was not associated with right colon diverticulitis [97]. As methanogen density is higher in the left colon [15], an increase in methane production that reduced transit time and increased intraluminal pressure would seem to be a contributing factor to the development of left colon diverticulitis.

7. Mitigation strategies

IBS is the most common functional gastrointestinal disorder and affects up to 12–15% of adults in the United States. Roughly 1.6 million Americans currently suffer with CD or UC, collectively known as IBD. IBS adversely impacts quality of life and medical expenditures, with significant costs arising from health-care visits and reduced workplace productivity, while IBD is a chronic, relapsing, debilitating disease associated with both environmental and genetic factors. IBD affects one in 200 Americans (80,000 children) at an estimated direct cost of $1.84 billion dollars. Conventional therapy attempts to modulate the immune response in the gut as it relates to IBD, yet many individuals continue to require surgery to control their disease or address its complications. There is a longstanding belief that dysbiosis (altered microbial environment) in the GIT plays an important etiologic role in the pathogenesis of IBS and IBD. There is significant scientific and public interest in compositional understanding of the intestinal microbiome (the specific constellation of microorganisms populating the gut) to better understand the role of the microbiome in health and disease. The contribution of individual organisms, including archaea, in the pathogenesis of GI disease is complex because of the rudimentary understanding of the compositional components of the microbiome.

The control of methanogen populations has long been a strategy in livestock to improve animal dietary efficiency, as methane production is an energy sink, as well as to reduce greenhouse gas emissions. In ruminant livestock, as discussed in a review by Hook et al. [24], this is largely done by manipulating the diet to improve the digestibility of feed and increase passage rate through the digestive tract to both deprive methanogens of potential precursors and to manually flush them out of the system. A change in diet is a potential avenue for reducing methanogen populations in humans, as methanogenesis is associated with sugar-/starch-based diets in monogastrics [27]. Environmental effects may also play a role, as children living near landfills, which had higher atmospheric methane than areas away from landfills, had a higher breath methane output and higher *Mbr. smithii* cell density than control children, regardless of their socioeconomic level [34]. Previous to that study, it was shown that the bacterial and fungal counts dispersed from landfills into air were up to 20 times higher than microbial counts from other areas [98].

Antibiotics have commonly been used to treat gastrointestinal disease or symptoms such as fasting and OGTT (glucose) levels [54], endotoxinemia and cecal LPS concentrations [51, 55], or global IBS symptoms [99]. Archaea are largely resistant to antimicrobial agents, which target bacteria, as they have different cell wall components and structure, and the few antimicrobials which they are susceptible to have been summarized in a recent review [100]. Notably, *Methanobrevibacter* species have only been shown to be susceptible to mevastatin and levastatin, both hydroxymethylglutaryl (HMG)-SCoA reductase inhibitors [101].

Our increasing knowledge of the potential long-term effects on gut microbial diversity has led to a trend of alternative treatments or mitigating methods over antibiotics. A recent review of probiotics showed them to be effective in relieving digestive dysbiosis symptoms or treating gastrointestinal conditions [79, 81, 102, 103]. The use of prebiotics directly infused into the colon, such as short-chain fatty acids, however, did not increase colonic motility [104]. While probiotics and other dietary additives have been used to reduce methanogenesis in ruminant livestock [24], the effect of probiotics on methanogen populations in humans has not yet been investigated. While current research suggests that methanogens and methane production may exacerbate symptoms, causative relations have only been shown in bacteria, and thus it is bacteria which should be the ultimate target for mitigation strategies in unhealthy populations.

Direct microbial remediation and mitigation have only been recently considered in human medicine with the advent of fecal transfer treatments from healthy donors. While this has mainly been aimed at remediating pathogenic bacterial populations, the implications for this technology to reduce methanogenesis and improve gastrointestinal conditions are clear. It may be possible to use fecal transfer treatments to increase the diversity of GIT archaea and thus promote competition to reduce methane production, to colonize with less-efficient methanogens, or to potentially increase competition by increasing SRB populations, which may have its own health implications for detoxifying hydrogen sulfate gas. Most interestingly, the transfer of fecal microbiota or cultures of specific methanogens has shown to also induce metabolic states in the recipients; fecal transfers, or colonization from parent to child, from overweight or pregnant individuals has been shown to increase weight gain in recipients [10, 16, 48, 105, 106]. While the possibility of this transfer to improve weight gain in severely malnourished individuals remains possible but not yet clinically applied, the more commercially appealing treatment of obesity using fecal transfers from lean individuals has yet to be explored.

8. Summary

Methane has been implicated in a number of gastrointestinal diseases, but methanogens have not yet been identified as causative agents. More work is needed in order to understand the interactions between archaea and host epithelia, as well as whether the root dysbiosis is caused by bacteria, archaea, or host epithelia. In addition, more sensitive, quick, and minimally invasive assessment techniques are needed to assess methane production, methanogen diversity, and methanogen density. In cases where methanogens are potentially pathogenic, more data are required to develop therapeutic antimicrobials or other mitigation strategies.

Author details

Suzanne L. Ishaq[1*], Peter L. Moses[2] and André-Denis G. Wright[3]

*Address all correspondence to: suzanne.pellegrini@montana.edu

1 Department of Animal and Range Sciences, Montana State University, Bozeman, USA

2 University of Vermont, College of Medicine, Burlington, USA

3 Department of Animal and Comparative Biomedical Sciences, University of Arizona, Tucson, USA

References

[1] Moses PL, Ishaq SL, Gupta K, Mauer SM, Wright A-DG: Biodiversity of human gut methanogens varies with concentration of exhaled breath methane. In Am Coll Gastroenterol 80th Annu Meet. Honolulu: American College of Gastroenterology; 2015: P776.

[2] Dridi B, Henry M, El Khéchine A, Raoult D, Drancourt M: High prevalence of Methanobrevibacter smithii and Methanosphaera stadtmanae detected in the human gut using an improved DNA detection protocol. PLoS One 2009, 4:e7063.

[3] Samuel BS, Hansen EE, Manchester JK, Coutinho PM, Henrissat B, Fulton R, Latreille P, Kim K, Wilson RK, Gordon JI: Genomic and metabolic adaptations of Methanobrevibacter smithii to the human gut. Proc Natl Acad Sci USA 2007, 104:10643–10648.

[4] Dridi B, Henry M, Richet H, Raoult D, Drancourt M: Age-related prevalence of Methanomassiliicoccus luminyensis in the human gut microbiome. APMIS 2012, 120:773–777.

[5] Fricke WF, Seedorf H, Henne A, Krüer M, Liesegang H, Hedderich R, Gottschalk G, Thauer RK: The genome sequence of Methanosphaera stadtmanae reveals why this human intestinal archaeon is restricted to methanol and H2 for methane formation and ATP synthesis. J Bacteriol 2006, 188:642–658.

[6] Levitt MD, Bond JH: Volume, composition, and source of intestinal gas. Gastroenterology 1970, 59:921–929.

[7] Zhou M, Hernandez-Sanabria E, Guan LL: Characterization of variation in rumen methanogenic communities under different dietary and host feed efficiency conditions, as determined by PCR-denaturing gradient gel electrophoresis analysis. Appl Environ Microbiol 2010, 76:3776–3786.

[8] Hoffmann C, Dollive S, Grunberg S, Chen J, Li H, Wu GD, Lewis JD, Bushman FD: Archaea and fungi of the human gut microbiome: correlations with diet and bacterial residents. PLoS One 2013, 8:e66019.

[9] Carberry CA, Waters SM, Kenny DA, Creevey CJ: Rumen methanogenic genotypes differ in abundance according to host residual feed intake phenotype and diet type. Appl Envir Microbiol 2014, 80:586–594.

[10] Samuel BS, Gordon JI: A humanized gnotobiotic mouse model of host-archaeal-bacterial mutualism. Proc Natl Acad Sci USA 2006, 103:10011–10016.

[11] Joblin KN, Naylor GE, Williams AG: Effect of Methanobrevibacter smithii on xylanolytic activity of anaerobic ruminal fungi. Appl Envir Microbiol 1990, 56:2287–2295.

[12] Facey H V, Northwood KS, Wright A-DG: Molecular diversity of methanogens in fecal samples from captive Sumatran orangutans (Pongo abelii). Amer J Primatol 2012, 74:408–413.

[13] Jones WJ, Nagle DP, Whitman WB: Methanogens and the diversity of archaebacteria. Microbiol Rev 1987, 51:135–177.

[14] Thomas NA, Jarrell KF: Characterization of flagellum gene families of methanogenic archaea and localization of novel flagellum accessory proteins. J Bacteriol 2001, 183:7154–7164.

[15] Flourie B, Etanchaud F, Florent C, Pellier P, Bouhnik Y, Rambaud JC: Comparative study of hydrogen and methane production in the human colon using caecal and faecal homogenates. Gut 1990, 31:684–685.

[16] Mathur R, Kim G, Morales W, Sung J, Rooks E, Pokkunuri V, Weitsman S, Barlow GM, Chang C, Pimentel M: Intestinal Methanobrevibacter smithii but not total bacteria is related to diet-induced weight gain in rats. Obesity (Silver Spring) 2013, 21:748–754.

[17] Horz H-P, Conrads G: Methanogenic archaea and oral infections—ways to unravel the black box. J Oral Microbiol 2011, 3:1–11.

[18] Maukonen J, Mättö J, Suihko M-L, Saarela M: Intra-individual diversity and similarity of salivary and faecal microbiota. J Med Microbiol 2008, 57(Pt 12):1560–1568.

[19] Cloarec D, Bornet F, Gouilloud S, Barry JL, Salim B, Galmiche JP: Breath hydrogen response to lactulose in healthy subjects: relationship to methane producing status. Gut 1990, 31:300–304.

[20] Jahng J, Jung IS, Choi EJ, Conklin JL, Park H: The effects of methane and hydrogen gases produced by enteric bacteria on ileal motility and colonic transit time. Neurogastroenterol Motil 2012, 24:185–190, e92.

[21] Ohsawa I, Ishikawa M, Takahashi K, Watanabe M, Nishimaki K, Yamagata K, Katsura K-I, Katayama Y, Asoh S, Ohta S: Hydrogen acts as a therapeutic antioxidant by selectively reducing cytotoxic oxygen radicals. Nat Med 2007, 13:688–694.

[22] Ohta S: Recent progress toward hydrogen medicine: potential of molecular hydrogen for preventive and therapeutic applications. Curr Pharm Des 2011, 17:2241–2252.

[23] Janssen PH: Influence of hydrogen on rumen methane formation and fermentation balances through microbial growth kinetics and fermentation thermodynamics. Anim Feed Sci Technol 2010, 160:1–22.

[24] Hook SE, Wright A-DG, McBride BW: Methanogens: methane producers of the rumen and mitigation strategies. Archaea 2010, 2010:945785.

[25] Issa R: Non-pathogenic protozoa. Int J Pharma Pharm Sci 2014, 6:30–40.

[26] Molecular Detection of Human Parasitic Pathogens. Dongyou Liu, editor. New York: CRC Press; 2012, 895 p. ISBN: 978-1-4398-1242-6

[27] Christl SU, Murgatroyd PR, Gibson GR, Cummings JH: Production, metabolism, and excretion of hydrogen in the large intestine. Gastroenterology 1992, 102(4 Pt 1):1269–1277.

[28] Zhang Y, Tang Z-H, Ren Z, Qu S-L, Liu M-H, Liu L-S, Jiang Z-S: Hydrogen sulfide, the next potent preventive and therapeutic agent in aging and age-associated diseases. Mol Cell Biol 2013, 33:1104–1113.

[29] Cord-Ruwisch R, Seitz H-J, Conrad R: The capacity of hydrogentrophic anaerobic bacteria to compete for traces of hydrogen depends on the redox potential of the electron acceptor. Arch Microbiol 1988, 149:350–357.

[30] Lopez S, McIntosh FM, Wallace RJ, Newbold CJ: Effect of adding acetogenic bacteria on methane production by mixed rumen microorganisms. Anim Feed Sci Technol 1999, 78:1–9.

[31] Sahakian AB, Jee S-R, Pimentel M: Methane and the gastrointestinal tract. Dig Dis Sci 2010, 55:2135–2143.

[32] Kormas KA, Meziti A, Mente E, Frentzos A: Dietary differences are reflected on the gut prokaryotic community structure of wild and commercially reared sea bream (Sparus aurata). Microbiologyopen 2014, 3:718–728.

[33] Weaver GA, Krause JA, Miller TL, Wolin MJ: Incidence of methanogenic bacteria in a sigmoidoscopy population: an association of methanogenic bacteria and diverticulosis. Gut 1986, 27:698–704.

[34] de Araujo Filho HB, Carmo-Rodrigues MS, Mello CS, Melli LCFL, Tahan S, Pignatari ACC, de Morais MB: Children living near a sanitary landfill have increased breath methane and Methanobrevibacter smithii in their intestinal microbiota. Archaea 2014, 2014:576249.

[35] McKay LF, Eastwood MA, Brydon WC: Methane excretion in man—a study of breath, flatus, and faeces. Gut 1985, 26:69–74.

[36] Pimentel M, Lin HC, Enayati P, van den Burg B, Lee H-R, Chen JH, Park S, Kong Y, Conklin J: Methane, a gas produced by enteric bacteria, slows intestinal transit and augments small intestinal contractile activity. Am J Physiol Gastrointest Liver Physiol 2006, 290:G1089–G1095.

[37] Wang R: Two's company, three's a crowd: can H2S be the third endogenous gaseous transmitter? FASEB J 2002, 16:1792–1798.

[38] Ignarro LJ, Buga GM, Wood KS, Byrns RE, Chaudhuri G: Endothelium-derived relaxing factor produced and released from artery and vein is nitric oxide. Proc Natl Acad Sci 1987, 84:9265–9269.

[39] Haines A, Metz G, Dilawari J, Blendis L, Wiggins H: Breath-methane in patients with cancer of the large bowel. Lancet (London, England) 1977, 2:481–483.

[40] Rana SV, Malik A: Breath tests and irritable bowel syndrome. World J Gastroenterol 2014, 20:7587–7601.

[41] Mathur R, Amichai M, Chua KS, Mirocha J, Barlow GM, Pimentel M: Methane and hydrogen positivity on breath test is associated with greater body mass index and body fat. J Clin Endocrinol Metab 2013, 98:E698–E702.

[42] Pimentel M, Mayer AG, Park S, Chow EJ, Hasan A, Kong Y: Methane production during lactulose breath test is associated with gastrointestinal disease presentation. Dig Dis Sci 2003, 48:86–92.

[43] Drossman DA: The functional gastrointestinal disorders and the Rome III process. Gastroenterol 2006, 130:1377–1390.

[44] Ley RE, Bäckhed F, Turnbaugh PJ, Lozupone CA, Knight RD, Gordon JI: Obesity alters gut microbial ecology. Proc Natl Acad Sci USA 2005, 102:11070–11075.

[45] Tsai Y-T, Cheng P-C, Pan T-M: Anti-obesity effects of gut microbiota are associated with lactic acid bacteria. Appl Microbiol Biotech 2013, 1:1–10.

[46] Turnbaugh PJ, Hamady M, Yatsunenko T, Cantarel BL, Duncan AE, Ley RE, Sogin ML, Jones WJ, Roe BA, Affourtit JP, Egholm M, Henrissat B, Heath AC, Knight R, Gordon JI: A core gut microbiome in obese and lean twins. Nature 2009, 457:480–484.

[47] Turnbaugh PJ, Ley RE, Mahowald MA, Magrini V, Mardis ER, Gordon JI: An obesity-associated gut microbiome with increased capacity for energy harvest. Nature 2006, 444:424–438.

[48] Koren O, Goodrich JK, Cullender TC, Spor A, Laitinen K, Bäckhed HK, Gonzalez A, Werner JJ, Angenent LT, Knight R, Bäckhed F, Isolauri E, Salminen S, Ley RE: Host remodeling of the gut microbiome and metabolic changes during pregnancy. Cell 2012, 150:470–480.

[49] Bäckhed F, Ding H, Wang T, Hooper L V, Koh GY, Nagy A, Semenkovich CF, Gordon JI: The gut microbiota as an environmental factor that regulates fat storage. Proc Natl Acad Sci USA 2004, 101:15718–15723.

[50] Vijay-Kumar M, Aitken JD, Carvalho FA, Cullender TC, Mwangi S, Srinivasan S, Sitaraman S V, Knight R, Ley RE, Gewirtz AT: Metabolic syndrome and altered gut microbiota in mice lacking Toll-like receptor 5. Science 2010, 328:228–231.

[51] Cani PD, Bibiloni R, Knauf C, Waget A, Neyrinck AM, Delzenne NM, Burcelin R: Changes in gut microbiota control metabolic endotoxemia-induced inflammation in high-fat diet-induced obesity and diabetes in mice. Diabetes 2008, 57:1470–1481.

[52] Creely SJ, McTernan PG, Kusminski CM, Fisher fM, Da Silva NF, Khanolkar M, Evans M, Harte AL, Kumar S: Lipopolysaccharide activates an innate immune system response in human adipose tissue in obesity and type 2 diabetes. Am J Physiol Endocrinol Metab 2007, 292:E740–E747.

[53] Cani PD, Amar J, Iglesias MA, Poggi M, Knauf C, Bastelica D, Neyrinck AM, Fava F, Tuohy KM, Chabo C, Waget A, Delmée E, Cousin B, Sulpice T, Chamontin B, Ferrières J, Tanti J-F, Gibson GR, Casteilla L, Delzenne NM, Alessi MC, Burcelin R: Metabolic endotoxemia initiates obesity and insulin resistance. Diabetes 2007, 56:1761–1772.

[54] Musso G, Gambino R, Cassader M: Obesity, diabetes, and gut microbiota: the hygiene hypothesis expanded? Diabetes Care 2010, 33:2277–2284.

[55] Chou CJ, Membrez M, Blancher F: Gut decontamination with norfloxacin and ampicillin enhances insulin sensitivity in mice. Nestlé Nutr Work Ser Paediatr Program 2008, 62:127–140.

[56] Basseri RJ, Basseri B, Pimentel M, Chong K, Youdim A, Low K, Hwang L, Soffer E, Chang C, Mathur R: Intestinal methane production in obese individuals is associated with a higher body mass index. Gastroenterol Hepatol (N Y) 2012, 8:22–28.

[57] Armougom F, Henry M, Vialettes B, Raccah D, Raoult D: Monitoring bacterial community of human gut microbiota reveals an increase in Lactobacillus in obese patients and methanogens in anorexic patients. PLoS One 2009, 4:e7125.

[58] Faria M, Pavin EJ, Parisi MCR, Lorena SLS, Brunetto SQ, Ramos CD, Pavan CR, Mesquita MA: Delayed small intestinal transit in patients with long-standing type 1 diabetes mellitus: investigation of the relationships with clinical features, gastric emptying, psychological distress, and nutritional parameters. Diabetes Technol Ther 2013, 15:32–38.

[59] Cesario V, Di Rienzo TA, Campanale M, D'angelo G, Barbaro F, Gigante G, Vitale G, Scavone G, Pitocco D, Gasbarrini A, Ojetti V: Methane intestinal production and poor metabolic control in type I diabetes complicated by autonomic neuropathy. Minerva Endocrinol 2014, 39:201–207.

[60] Ojetti V, Pitocco D, Scarpellini E, Zaccardi F, Scaldaferri F, Gigante G, Gasbarrini G, Ghirlanda G, Gasbarrini A: Small bowel bacterial overgrowth and type 1 diabetes. Eur Rev Med Pharmacol Sci 2009, 13:419–423.

[61] Mathur R, Goyal D, Kim G, Barlow GM, Chua KS, Pimentel M: Methane-producing human subjects have higher serum glucose levels during oral glucose challenge than non-methane producers: a pilot study of the effects of enteric methanogens on glycemic regulation. Res J Endocrinol Metab 2014, 2.

[62] American Cancer Society. 2016. Accessed March 10, 2016. Available from: www.cancer.org

[63] Mazmanian SK, Liu CH, Tzianabos AO, Kasper DL: An immunomodulatory molecule of symbiotic bacteria directs maturation of the host immune system. Cell 2005, 122:107–118.

[64] Xuan C, Shamonki JM, Chung A, Dinome ML, Chung M, Sieling PA, Lee DJ: Microbial dysbiosis is associated with human breast cancer. PLoS One 2014, 9:e83744.

[65] Blaser MJ: Understanding microbe-induced cancers. Cancer Prev Res (Phila) 2008, 1:15–20.

[66] Eckburg PB, Lepp PW, Relman DA: Archaea and their potential role in human disease. Infect Immun 2003, 71:591–596.

[67] Gill EE, Brinkman FSL: The proportional lack of archaeal pathogens: do viruses/phages hold the key? Bioessays 2011, 33:248–254.

[68] Roccarina D, Lauritano EC, Gabrielli M, Franceschi F, Ojetti V, Gasbarrini A: The role of methane in intestinal diseases. Am J Gastroenterol 2010, 105:1250–1256.

[69] Scanlan PD, Shanahan F, Marchesi JR: Human methanogen diversity and incidence in healthy and diseased colonic groups using mcrA gene analysis. BMC Microbiol 2008, 8:79.

[70] Abell GCJ, Conlon Ma, McOrist AL: Methanogenic archaea in adult human faecal samples are inversely related to butyrate concentration. Microb Ecol Health Dis 2006, 18(September):154–160.

[71] Kim YS, Milner JA: Dietary modulation of colon cancer risk. J Nutr 2007, 137(11 Suppl): 2576S–2579S.

[72] Smith CJ, Rocha ER, Pastor BJ: The medically important Bacteroides spp. in health and disease. Prokaryotes 2006, 7:381–427.

[73] Scheppach W: Effects of short chain fatty acids on gut morphology and function. Gut 1994, 35(1 Suppl):S35–S38.

[74] Piqué JM, Pallarés M, Cusó E, Vilar-Bonet J, Gassull MA: Methane production and colon cancer. Gastroenterology 1984, 87:601–605.

[75] Holma R, Korpela R, Sairanen U, Blom M, Rautio M, Poussa T, Saxelin M, Osterlund P: Colonic methane production modifies gastrointestinal toxicity associated with adjuvant 5-fluorouracil chemotherapy for colorectal cancer. J Clin Gastroenterol 2013, 47:45–51.

[76] Liebling T, Rosenman KD, Pastides H, Griffith RG, Lemeshow S: Cancer mortality among workers exposed to formaldehyde. Am J Ind Med 1984, 5:423–428.

[77] Attene-Ramos MS, Wagner ED, Plewa MJ, Gaskins HR: Evidence that hydrogen sulfide is a genotoxic agent. Mol Cancer Res 2006, 4:9–14.

[78] Szabo C, Coletta C, Chao C, Módis K, Szczesny B, Papapetropoulos A, Hellmich MR: Tumor-derived hydrogen sulfide, produced by cystathionine-β-synthase, stimulates bioenergetics, cell proliferation, and angiogenesis in colon cancer. Proc Natl Acad Sci USA 2013, 110:12474–12479.

[79] Aragon G, Graham DB, Borum M, Doman DB: Probiotic therapy for irritable bowel syndrome. Gastroenterol Hepatol (N Y) 2010, 6:39–44.

[80] Xu G-Y, Winston JH, Shenoy M, Zhou S, Chen JDZ, Pasricha PJ: The endogenous hydrogen sulfide producing enzyme cystathionine-beta synthase contributes to visceral hypersensitivity in a rat model of irritable bowel syndrome. Mol Pain 2009, 5:44.

[81] Maccaferri S, Candela M, Turroni S, Centanni M, Severgnini M, Consolandi C, Cavina P, Brigidi P: IBS-associated phylogenetic unbalances of the intestinal microbiota are not reverted by probiotic supplementation. Gut Microbes 2012, 3:406–413.

[82] Saulnier DM, Riehle K, Mistretta T-A, Diaz M-A, Mandal D, Raza S, Weidler EM, Qin X, Coarfa C, Milosavljevic A, Petrosino JF, Highlander S, Gibbs R, Lynch S V, Shulman RJ, Versalovic J: Gastrointestinal microbiome signatures of pediatric patients with irritable bowel syndrome. Gastroenterology 2011, 141:1782–1791.

[83] Nelson TA, Holmes S, Alekseyenko A V, Shenoy M, DeSantis TZ, Wu CH, Andersen GL, Winston J, Sonnenburg J, Pasricha PJ, Spormann A: PhyloChip microarray analysis reveals altered gastrointestinal microbial communities in a rat model of colonic hypersensitivity. Neurogastroenterol and Motil 2011, 23:169–177, e41–2.

[84] Kumar S, Misra A, Ghoshal UC: Patients with irritable bowel syndrome exhale more hydrogen than healthy subjects in fasting state. J Neurogastroenterol Motil 2010, 16:299–305.

[85] Furnari M, Savarino E, Bruzzone L, Moscatelli A, Gemignani L, Giannini EG, Zentilin P, Dulbecco P, Savarino V: Reassessment of the role of methane production between irritable bowel syndrome and functional constipation. J Gastroenterol Liver Dis 2012, 21:157–163.

[86] Mann NS, Limoges-Gonzales M: The prevalence of small intestinal bacterial overgrowth in irritable bowel syndrome. Hepatogastroenterology 2009, 56:718–721.

[87] Magge S, Lembo A: Low-FODMAP diet for treatment of irritable bowel syndrome. Gastroenterol Hepatol (N Y) 2012, 8:739–745.

[88] Simrén M, Månsson A, Langkilde AM, Svedlund J, Abrahamsson H, Bengtsson U, Björnsson ES: Food-related gastrointestinal symptoms in the irritable bowel syndrome. Digestion 2001, 63:108–115.

[89] Zhu Y, Zheng X, Cong Y, Chu H, Fried M, Dai N, Fox M: Bloating and distention in irritable bowel syndrome: the role of gas production and visceral sensation after lactose ingestion in a population with lactase deficiency. Am J Gastroenterol 2013, 108:1516–1525.

[90] Kim G, Deepinder F, Morales W, Hwang L, Weitsman S, Chang C, Gunsalus R, Pimentel M: Methanobrevibacter smithii is the predominant methanogen in patients with constipation-predominant IBS and methane on breath. Dig Dis Sci 2012, 57:3213–3218.

[91] Rajilić-Stojanović M, Heilig HGHJ, Molenaar D, Kajander K, Surakka A, Smidt H, de Vos WM: Development and application of the human intestinal tract chip, a phylogenetic microarray: analysis of universally conserved phylotypes in the abundant microbiota of young and elderly adults. Env Microbiol 2009, 11:1736–1751.

[92] Blais Lecours P, Duchaine C, Taillefer M, Tremblay C, Veillette M, Cormier Y, Marsolais D: Immunogenic properties of archaeal species found in bioaerosols. PLoS One 2011, 6:e23326.

[93] Blais Lecours P, Marsolais D, Cormier Y, Berberi M, Haché C, Bourdages R, Duchaine C: Increased prevalence of Methanosphaera stadtmanae in inflammatory bowel diseases. PLoS One 2014, 9:e87734.

[94] Paun A, Danska JS: Immuno-ecology: how the microbiome regulates tolerance and autoimmunity. Curr Opin Immunol 2015, 37:34–39.

[95] Attaluri A, Jackson M, Valestin J, Rao SSC: Methanogenic flora is associated with altered colonic transit but not stool characteristics in constipation without IBS. Amer J Gastroenterol 2010, 105:1407–1411.

[96] Painter NS, Burkitt DP: Diverticular disease of the colon: a deficiency disease of Western civilization. Br Med J 1971, 2:450–454.

[97] Jang S-I, Kim J-H, Youn YH, Park H, Lee SI, Conklin JL: Relationship between intestinal gas and the development of right colonic diverticula. J Neurogastroenterol Motil 2010, 16:418–423.

[98] Rahkonen P, Ettala M, Laukkanen M, Salkinoja-Salonen M: Airborne microbes and endotoxins in the work environment of two sanitary landfills in Finland. Aerosol Sci Technol 1990, 13:505–513.

[99] Pimentel M, Lembo A, Chey WD, Zakko S, Ringel Y, Yu J, Mareya SM, Shaw AL, Bortey E, Forbes WP: Rifaximin therapy for patients with irritable bowel syndrome without constipation. New Eng J Med 2011, 364:22–32.

[100] Pimentel M, Gunsalus RP, Rao SSC, Zhang H: Methanogens in human health and disease. Amer J Gastroenterol 2012, 1:28–33.

[101] Miller TL, Wolin MJ: Methanogens in human and animal intestinal tracts. Syst Appl Microbiol 1986, 7:223–229.

[102] Choi CH, Chang SK: Alteration of gut microbiota and efficacy of probiotics in functional constipation. J Neurogastroenterol Motil 2015, 21:4–7.

[103] Ringel Y, Quigley EM, Lin HC: Using probiotics in gastrointestinal disorders. Amer J Gastroenterol Suppl 2012, 1:34–40.

[104] Jouët P, Moussata D, Duboc H, Boschetti G, Attar A, Gorbatchef C, Sabaté J-M, Coffin B, Flourié B: Effect of short-chain fatty acids and acidification on the phasic and tonic motor activity of the human colon. Neurogastroenterol Motil 2013, 25:943–949.

[105] Alang N, Kelly CR: Weight gain after fecal microbiota transplantation. Open Forum Infect Dis 2015, 2:ofv004.

[106] Ridaura VK, Faith JJ, Rey FE, Cheng J, Duncan AE, Kau AL, Griffin NW, Lombard V, Henrissat B, Bain JR, Muehlbauer MJ, Ilkayeva O, Semenkovich CF, Funai K, Hayashi DK, Lyle BJ, Martini MC, Ursell LK, Clemente JC, Van Treuren W, Walters WA, Knight R, Newgard CB, Heath AC, Gordon JI: Gut microbiota from twins discordant for obesity modulate metabolism in mice. Science 2013, 341:1241214.

Section 3

Gut Dysberiosis on the Human Brain

Chapter 3

Consequences of Gut Dysbiosis on the Human Brain

Richard A. Hickman, Maryem A. Hussein and
Zhiheng Pei

Additional information is available at the end of the chapter

http://dx.doi.org/10.5772/64690

Abstract

The central nervous system (CNS) and the gastrointestinal (GI) tract develop in parallel and communicate with each other throughout life using neural, endocrine, and immune pathways, giving rise to the concept of a 'gut-brain axis' in which both organ systems intimately interact. Fundamental to the axis is the GI microbiome, which is the collective genomic aggregate of bacteria and other microorganisms that dwell within the lumen of the GI tract. Increasing evidence gathered from animal models and human studies demonstrates that perturbation of the microbiome, otherwise known as dysbiosis, can lead to specific neurological and psychiatric disorders. This chapter will provide a brief review of the literature that reveals the influence of the microbiome in CNS disease and provide perspectives in treatment through modification of the microbiome.

Keywords: microbiome, dysbiosis, brain, multiple sclerosis, Parkinson's disease

1. Introduction to the brain-gut-microbiome axis

The human microbiome has emerged as an entity with a tremendous degree of influence in health and disease.[1] Bacteria within the GI tract perform a wide range of symbiotic functions for their host, which range from digestion and the production of bioactive metabolites to influencing the healthy development and function of the immune system [1, 2]. All of these local effects on the GI tract have the ability to impact the brain through neural connections,

[1] For the purposes of this chapter, the microbiome mentioned herein refers to the combined aggregate of bacteria, viruses, fungi, archaea, and protista.

INTECH
open science | open minds

© 2016 The Author(s). Licensee InTech. This chapter is distributed under the terms of the Creative Commons Attribution License (http://creativecommons.org/licenses/by/3.0), which permits unrestricted use, distribution, and reproduction in any medium, provided the original work is properly cited. (cc) BY

such as the vagus nerve, and by endocrine means [3, 4]. The awareness of this two-way interaction between the gut and the brain has now provided more explanations for some conditions otherwise labeled as 'functional disorders' and has also laid fertile ground for the discovery of new treatment modalities in modulating the microbiome in treating CNS disease [5–7].

Significant development of the microbiome begins at the time of delivery. Vaginally, born infants are colonized by maternal fecal and vaginal microorganisms, whilst those born by Cesarean section are colonized by skin flora [8, 9]. Although the dogma has been that the antenatal intrauterine environment is sterile, this notion has been challenged by several findings, most notably that meconium contains bacterial colonies. Therefore, this implies that the influence of the microbiome may extend into the prenatal period [10, 11]. Following birth, the microbiome adapts according to factors such as dietary intake, antibiotic use, and living conditions. As the CNS and microbiome develop in parallel, significant changes in the microbiota occur at critical neurodevelopment time periods [12, 13]. Disruptions in the evolutionary progression of the microbiome may therefore have a lasting impact on the healthy development of the brain and *vice versa* because of this close interaction between the two systems.

The term 'dysbiosis' refers to an imbalance of microorganisms within the mucosal flora. Hepatic encephalopathy is the archetypal example of how a GI dysbiosis can result in CNS damage. Liver cirrhosis results in a distinct microbiota signature that differs significantly from healthy, control subjects [14]. Accumulation of toxic mediators, such as ammonium produced by urease-producing bacteria, enters the portal circulation. Blood ammonium concentrations rise, cross the blood-brain barrier, and accumulate within the brain leading to astrocytic damage and cerebral edema [15–17]. Curiously, however, treatment with the oral antibiotic rifaximin does not cause clinical improvement through changing the proportions of bacteria in the microbiome, but rather, the improvement in endotoxemia and cognition appears to be through modulation of bacterial metabolism [18–21]. Therefore, derangements of the microbiome that result in CNS dysfunction are not limited to constitutional changes but may also be influenced by its metabolic activity.

2. The influence of the microbiome in multiple sclerosis

2.1. Epidemiology and pathogenesis

Multiple sclerosis (MS) is the most common CNS demyelinating disease and is classically depicted by the acquisition of discrete demyelinating plaques within the grey and white matter of the CNS [22–24]. The acute MS plaque is characterized by infiltration of inflammatory cells with concomitant demyelination and edema [25]. Perivascular lymphocytic cuffing comprised predominantly of T cells is seen. There is a reactive astrogliosis with variable amounts of oligodendrocyte apoptosis within the plaque [26]. Over time, the plaques become sclerotic, representing the final pathological event at that location after a period of marked inflammation, astrogliosis, demyelination, remyelination, and axonal loss.

Despite this common pathological hallmark of the disease, MS is remarkably heterogeneous in terms of clinical presentation and prognosis [27]. Furthermore, the exact pathogenesis still remains poorly understood, although it is clear that both genetics and the environment have significant influences in the onset of MS and a complex interplay exists between these elements [28, 29]. Certainly, inflammation plays a key role in the pathophysiology of the disease. Most researchers favor an autoimmune hypothesis whereby autoreactive immune cells targeting myelin antigens are activated, likely incited by an environmental trigger [30].

Migrational studies have provided insight into how environmental changes may influence the risk of development of MS. Generally, populations further away from the equator have an increased risk of developing MS than those closer to the equator [31, 32]. Many studies have demonstrated that people migrating from high-risk areas to low-risk areas can be at sustained risk if the migration occurred after a certain critical age point [33]. Conversely, if the age of migration is younger than the critical age point, the individual is conferred the risk of the new region. The human microbiome is recognized to exhibit great geographical variation between populations and the local environment has a marked influence on the development of the microbiota [34, 35]. Given that the microbiota influences neurodevelopment and immunity early in life, one can speculate that this may explain why the conferred migrational risk of MS is age-dependent.

The first suggestion that MS may be related to hygienic living conditions was reported by Liebowitz et al. in 1966 [36]. By examining the degree of crowded living conditions, they found that the incidence of MS was higher in those that are more sanitary. The hygiene hypothesis, formulated later by Strachan in 1989, proposed that allergy and autoimmune diseases are, at least in part, the consequence of inadequate immune stimulation against pathogens during the early years of life that causes aberrant responses to self in later years [37, 38].

One MS epidemic occurred during the British occupation of the Faroe Islands during World War II. Prior to the arrival of British troops in 1940, there were no documented cases of MS in the native born Faroese on the islands. After 1943, there were four MS epidemics and the patients were located in proximity to the British encampments [39, 40]. The conclusion was that somehow the British troops had introduced an unknown pathogenic organism into the islands. Interestingly, the incidence of several infections increased during the occupation that coincided with MS epidemics, notably gastroenteritis and mumps infections, suggesting an association between MS and dysbiosis [41].

Aside from geographical predispositions for MS, other risk factors such as obesity, cigarette smoking, female sex, and low vitamin D levels are all associated with differences in the composition and/ or metabolic activity of the microbiota [42–49]. These epidemiological findings insinuate a potential role for the human microbiome in predisposing MS.

2.2. Bacterial dysbiosis and MS

Some of the initial indications that the GI microbiota may play a role in the pathogenesis of MS arose from work on experimental allergic encephalomyelitis (EAE) in germ-free (GF) mice. For decades, EAE has been used extensively as an animal model of demyelinating disease in which exposure to CNS myelin components, such as spinal cord homogenate or specific myelin proteins, triggers a T-cell-mediated autoimmune response that leads to CNS demyelination [50, 51]. Although there are similarities to relapsing remitting MS, there are notable differences that have been reviewed elsewhere (refer to Sriram and Steiner for a detailed review [50]).

Evidence that the gut microbiota can influence autoimmunity has been gathered from experiments that contrast conventionally housed animals with a normal composition of microbiota [also known as specific pathogen free (SPF) or conventionally colonized (CC)], and those maintained in a sterile environment [germ-free (GF) animals], thus removing the possibility of postnatal colonization of their GI tract. The absence of gut microbiota at birth affects the gut-associated lymphoid tissue (GALT), such that GF mice have hypoplastic Peyer's patches and mesenteric lymph nodes. Furthermore, the lymph nodes have fewer germinal centers and IgA-producing plasma cells than normally present in controls [49, 52]. Beyond the GI tract, the spleen and lymph nodes are also poorly developed [53]. This maldevelopment of the lymphoreticular system provides an explanation as to why GF mice are more prone to infection and why the risk of developing autoimmune disease is modified [54]. The gut microbiome has been shown to influence the probability of developing EAE in GF and SPF mice. Berer et al. showed that in SJL/J mice that have autoreactive CD4 T cells to myelin oligodendrocyte protein, the presence of the GI microbiota promoted the development of EAE [55]. Furthermore, the absence of GI microorganisms in GF mice and the consequent limited production of T_H17 cells within the GI tract and spleen appear to be protective against EAE unlike in controls [56, 57]. When segmented filamentous bacteria, which are known to induce the production of T_H17 cells, are inoculated into the GF mice, these animals developed EAE with antigenic stimulation, demonstrating that specific bacterial species within the gut microflora can predispose autoimmune demyelinating disease [56].

Several studies have demonstrated changes in the abundances of various bacterial taxa in MS compared with controls. Miyake et al. investigated fecal samples collected during the remission phase from patients with relapsing remitting MS and demonstrated 21 species that were significantly different in relative abundance [58]. Fourteen of these species belonged to the *Clostridia* clusters XIVa and IV, which were reduced in MS patients and are recognized to have an anti-inflammatory role [59]. Furthermore, *Bacteriodes* and *Prevotella* species were less prevalent in MS, although the exact pathogenic significance of this is yet defined. Of note, however, they did not discuss the possible confounding influence of medical therapy that may have been administered to these patients.

Rumah et al. identified *Clostridium perfringens* type B in the stool of a patient 3 months after the onset of MS symptoms [60]. *C. perfringens* B has the capability of producing Epsilon toxin (ETX), which can cross the blood-brain barrier and have toxicity to oligodendrocytes, thus providing a possible mechanism for demyelination in MS [61, 62]. Their analysis also revealed a reduced frequency of *C. perfringens* A in the GI tract of MS patients and that ETX reactivity was ten times more common than in controls. Another group identified a significantly increased Archaea (*Methanobrevibacteriaceae*) in MS contrasted with controls [63]. *Methanobrevibacter smithii* is considered to be strongly immunogenic and may be pro-inflammatory in the host. The same researchers also identified several organisms that were anti-inflammatory and were seen in a lower abundance in MS. Significant differences in microbiota in *Proteobacteria,* such as enrichment of *Shigella* and *Escherichia,* were also observed in pediatric MS when compared with controls [64].

2.3. Viral etiology

Many viruses have been implicated as risk factors for the development of MS [65]. Perhaps the most discussed has been the Epstein-Barr virus (EBV), which can be present in the oral microbiome and can be transmitted by saliva [66]. Humans are the obligate host for EBV and while many healthy controls are infected, nearly all patients with MS have seropositivity for EBV [67]. Furthermore, infectious mononucleosis (IM) resulting from EBV infection doubles the risk of developing MS. Similarly, a recent meta-analysis revealed significant associations between anti-EBNA (EBV nuclear antigen) IgG positivity, infectious mononucleosis, and smoking in conferring an increased risk of developing MS [68–70].

Several research findings have identified the presence of EBV within B cells from MS patients. One study identified the presence of EBV latent proteins being expressed in B cell follicles within the cerebral meninges and that the infiltrating B cells had EBV infection [71]. Interestingly, the cerebrospinal fluid (CSF) in MS is usually associated with oligoclonal bands, which is the product of IgG secretion from clonally expanded B cells [72]. Screening of these oligoclonal antibodies has identified BRRF2 and EBNA-1, which are EBV-related proteins, as possible targets of the CSF IgG immune response [73]. Exactly, how EBV fits into the pathogenesis of MS remains to be determined; however, its association with the oral microbiome in MS is evident.

2.4. Altering the microbiome-protection against MS by helminth infection

Certain helminthic infections appear to reduce the risk of developing MS [74]. Infection with *Trypanosoma cruzi* and *Paracoccidiodes brasiliensis* in MS patients causes lymphocytes to produce higher amounts of interleukin-10 (IL-10) and neurotrophic factors, such as brain-derived neurotrophic factor (BDNF) and nerve growth factor (NGF), in comparison with controls [75]. In MS, there is usually a low amount of IL-10 secretion favoring a T_H1 response, rather than a T_H2 response as is present in helminthic infections [76]. *Trichuris suis* is a helminth that has efficacy when administered orally in inflammatory bowel disease (IBD). Treatment with this helminth in MS is associated with elevated IL-4 and IL-10 as well as radiological improvements on MRI [77]. Another group demonstrated reduction in IFN-γ and IL-2 as well as an increase in IL-10 and IL-4 in secondary progressive MS following *Trichuris suis* administration, suggestive of a shift toward a T_H2 response [78]. In summary, therapeutic manipulation of the gut microbiome that favors an overall anti-inflammatory phenotype appears to have great promise in the treatment of MS. Further trial data are needed in this field to evaluate its efficacy and safety.

3. Parkinson's disease (PD)

PD typically manifests with bradykinesia, postural instability, and resting tremor that results from progressive neurodegeneration within the basal ganglia that is associated with abnormal α-synuclein accumulation and Lewy body formation [79, 80]. Until recently, it was thought that PD originated within the CNS, in which the pathological protein α-synuclein spread from the dorsal motor nucleus of the vagus to involve the basal ganglia and thenceforth the cerebral hemispheres [81]. However, the characteristic pathology has since been found in tissues outside of the CNS. Slow transit constipation is now well recognized to be a common finding that predates the motor symptoms in PD and can be present many years prior to diagnosis [82–84].

Findings from autopsy and surgical pathology studies have demonstrated the presence of phosphorylated α-synuclein in the sublingual glands and within Auerbach's and Meissner's plexuses of the enteric nervous system [85–87]. Consistent with these findings, GI pathology and concomitant symptoms predate motor features by at least 2 years [88, 89]. Transmission of α-synuclein from neuron to neuron has been elegantly shown in a rotenone animal model of PD wherein ingestion of rotenone causes release of α-synuclein and retrograde spread toward the brainstem; hemitransection of the vagal nerve, however, protects against ipsilateral synuclein pathology [90]. Similarly, neuronal transmission of α-synuclein occurs in human mesencephalic fetal transplants of PD patients in which α-synuclein is detected within the grafted cells at *postmortem* examination [91, 92]. The vagus nerve can therefore act as a conduit for the proteopathic spread of α-synuclein from the periphery to the brainstem. In a novel retrospective study, Svensson et al. showed a reduction in PD risk in patients who had truncal vagotomy compared with super-selective vagotomy and between truncal vagotomy and the general population [93]. While the study did not reach statistical significance, the complete severance of neural bidirectional communication between the GI tract and the brain may be beneficial in preventing the proteopathic spread of α-synuclein and hence avert PD neurodegeneration that might otherwise be inevitable.

Several pieces of data suggest that the microbiome has an involvement in PD. Scheperjans and colleagues demonstrated in a case control study of PD that *Prevotellaceae* species were significantly reduced whilst *Enterobacteriaceae* species were increased in patients with motor-predominant rather than tremor-predominant PD [94]. Furthermore, the quantity of *Enterobacteriaceae* correlated with the degree of postural instability. However, the question remains as to whether the dysbiosis is a consequence or cause of gastrointestinal dysmotility and also how this could influence the production, aggregation, or release of α-synuclein within the GI tract. Regardless of the microbiome's significance in the pathogenesis of PD, bacterial overgrowth that occurs in a proportion of patients with GI dysmotility can influence the symptomatic response to drug treatment. Malabsorption of drugs, in particular levodopa, is the probable reason for the increased motor fluctuations seen in this dysbiosis. Administration of rifaximin has shown improvement in these cases [95, 96].

The oral and nasal microbiota may also be relevant in PD and require investigation. The nucleus of the glossopharyngeal nerve exhibits α-synuclein deposits, and similarly to the vagus, the glossopharyngeal nerve may act as a route for peripheral entry of PD pathology into the brain. Furthermore, the olfactory bulb is frequently affected by PD pathology prior to the onset of motor symptoms and this is an explanation for the often prodromal anosmia [97]. Whether there is a dysbiosis in the oral or nasal cavity has yet to be ascertained, but may offer clues as to why PD pathology occurs in these other peripheral anatomic sites.

4. The role of the microbiome in psychiatric disease

The impact of the GI microbiome on human behavior and psychiatric disease is complex, but there are several observations that demonstrate strong associations between the two entities. First, anxiety and depression frequently co-exist with chronic gut disorders [98–102]. Second, mouse models of GI infection demonstrate elevated levels of anxiety-like behavior and alterations in CNS biochemistry [103]. Third, it was realized decades ago that stress occurring early in life or later in adulthood can alter the microbial composition of the gut [104]. More recent investigations conducted in animal models, and human patients have delved deeper into these associations and have attempted to elucidate how the commensal microbiome influences behavior.

The hypothalamic-pituitary-adrenal (HPA) axis is fundamental to the stress response, and endocrine disturbances of this axis have been attributed to depression and anxiety. In patients with severe depression, overactivation of the HPA axis causes hyper-secretion of catecholamines, corticotropin-releasing factor (CRF), and vasopressin [105]. Patients with depression often show elevated plasma cortisol levels, elevated CRF concentrations within the CSF and increased limbic concentrations of CRF [106, 107]. Sudo et al. conducted the first study to demonstrate the involvement of the gut microbiome in the normal development of the HPA axis [108]. GF mice were shown to have an exaggerated elevation of plasma adrenocorticotrophic hormone (ACTH) and corticosterone (the dominant glucocorticoid in rodents) in response to stress compared to SPF mice [108, 109]. However, when *Bifidobacterium infantis*, a bacterial species found in the infant gut, was inoculated in these mice, the exaggerated stress response was normalized. Importantly, this reversal took place only when the bacterial inoculation occurred by 6 weeks *postnatum*, suggesting a neurodevelopmental window of susceptibility to the effects of this bacteria-host interaction [108].

Other studies have focused on the effect of the microbiome on behavior and brain biochemistry. One of the challenges in interpreting the results of these reports is that they differ in animal strain, sex, and sourcing as well as overall experimental design. Despite these differences, it is clear that the microbiome influences both behavior and brain neurobiology. With regard to behavior, the majority of studies that compare GF with SPF mice report a decreased anxiety-like behavior in GF mice, in spite of an exaggerated HPA axis response to acute stress [109–111]. The one notable exception in mice, however, was a study by Nishino et al. [112]. This group compared GF mice with gnotobiotic mice, which are mice born in germ-free conditions to parents fed stools of SPF mice, and found that the ex-GF mice are less anxious. In this model, the transfer of the bacterial species *Brautia coccoides* reduces anxiety-like behavior [112].

Further evidence of the microbial influence on behavior derives from transferring microbiota between mouse strains of inherently different behavioral phenotypes. In a study by Bercik et al. colonization of GF mice with gut bacteria from donor mice with differing anxiety phenotypes transferred the behavioral phenotype of the donor to the recipient [113]. Again, it appears that there is a critical neurodevelopmental time point before which behavioral profiles are modifiable as adult GF mice colonized with SPF feces retain the anxiolytic behavioral phenotype of GF mice [110].

Animal studies that have investigated brain neurochemistry and examined monoamine concentrations and turnover rates have provided some insight into explaining these behavioral phenomena. Alterations in central monoamine neurotransmission, specifically serotonin (5-HT), norepinephrine (NE), and dopamine (DA), are known to play a role in anxiety and depression [114–119]. As would be predicted based on their behavioral patterns, ex-GF mice exhibit higher NE and DA turnover rates and have higher 5-HT concentrations in the striatum than their GF counterparts [112]. Furthermore, stress-sensitive rats that exhibit anxiety-like behavior when GF had a reduced DA turnover in the frontal cortex, striatum, and hippocampus than SPF rats [120]. Many of the studies that investigate monoamine transmission examine tryptophan levels as well, as tryptophan is required for the synthesis of 5-HT and may be low in depression [121]. Kynurenine, a metabolite of tryptophan, is increased in depression and the kynurenine:tryptophan ratio in blood correlates with anxiety [103, 122, 123]. Accordingly, the less anxious GF mice exhibit a decreased kynurenine:tryptophan ratio and increased plasma tryptophan concentrations compared to the more-anxious SPF mice [109]. In male GF mice, there is a significant sex-dependent increase in 5-HT and 5-hydroxyindoleacetic acid (5-HIAA) concentrations. Notably, the reduced anxiety seen in GF animals is normalized following microbial colonization as well as normalization of both the tryptophan concentrations and the kynurenine:tryptophan ratio. Interestingly, however, the increased 5-HT and 5-HIAA concentration in GF animals remains resistant to colonization [109]. Using mass spectrometry, Matsumoto et al. analyzed the cerebral metabolome of GF mice and ex-GF mice and identified 38 metabolites that differed significantly [124]. Notably, concentrations of DA were twofold higher in GF than in ex-GF mice; consistent with the findings that GF mice display increased motor activity and reduced anxiety-like behavior compared with their ex-GF counterparts. In the cerebrum of GF mice, the concentration of tryptophan was decreased but the study failed to find differences in 5-HT levels.

Various receptors, with known roles in depression and anxiety, are influenced by the microbiome. For instance, the 5HT1A receptor, which is associated with anxiety, has decreased expression in the dentate granule layer of the hippocampus in GF female mice [111]. The N-methyl-D-aspartate (NMDA) receptors are important for learning and memory. Sudo et al. reported downregulation in the NMDA receptor subunit 2A (NR2A) mRNA in the cortex and the hippocampus of GF mice compared to SPF mice [108]. Neufeld et al., however, did not detect differences in the hippocampal subregions by *in situ* hybridization but rather demonstrated a decrease in NMDA receptor subunit 2B (NR2B) mRNA expression in the central amygdala of GF mice [111]. Additionally, DA D1 receptor mRNA was significantly higher in the hippocampus of GF mice than in SPF mice [110].

In patients with depression, hippocampal neurogenesis is reduced along with levels of BDNF, and recent evidence indicates that increased hippocampal BDNF is associated with anxiolytic and antidepressant behavior [125]. In the studies of GF mice, the exact influence of the microbiome on BDNF is uncertain; some studies show increased hippocampal BDNF expression, while others show the opposite at both the mRNA and protein level. The differences in BDNF appear to be sex-related, with reductions in BDNF being observed mainly in male GF animals, and not in female animals [108, 109, 111]. Heijtz et al. showed that in GF mice, mRNA expression of nerve growth factor-inducible clone A (NGFI-A), implicated in the development of anxiety-like behavior, was significantly lower in the orbital frontal cortex, striatum, hippocampus, dentate gyrus, and amygdala compared with SPF mice [110]. These studies highlight a role for neurotrophic factors in the microbiome-gut-brain axis and its influence on anxiety and depression and further indicate that regulation of this axis may be sex dependent. The microbiome also appears to have a broader impact on neurobiology, as evidenced by a study looking at the amygdala that showed an altered transcriptome in GF compared to SPF mice. Specifically, in GF mice, there is upregulation of immediate early response genes with differential expression of genes involved in neurotransmission, plasticity, and metabolism [126].

4.1. Treatments that alter the microbial flora

4.1.1. Probiotics

Associations between the microbiome and behavior are reinforced by studies using probiotic therapy, which alter the gut microbial environment through the ingestion of live bacterial cultures. There is increasing evidence that certain strains are able to attenuate various behavioral and biochemical effects of stress. Adult rats given *Lactobacillus helveticus* NS8 display reduced stress-induced anxiety and depression that is comparable to citalopram therapy [127]. Biochemically, these rats had lower corticosterone and ACTH concentrations in the plasma, increased hippocampal monoamine concentrations and BDNF transcription as well as higher levels of plasma IL-10, which is an anti-inflammatory cytokine that is reduced in depressed patients [127]. Similarly, the probiotic formulation of *L. helveticus* R0052 and *B. longum* R0175 attenuated the response to chronic stress, with decreased levels of corticosterone, epinephrine, and NE within the plasma [128]. Furthermore, the probiotics *B. longum 1714* and *B. breve 1205* are anxiolytic in mice [129]. Probiotics with *B. infantis*, previously discussed as being capable of reversing the exaggerated stress response in GF mice, have shown various results in rats; one showed attenuation of behavioral and biochemical abnormalities associated with maternal separation, whilst another showed minimal behavioral effects, despite changes in the levels of various cytokines and metabolites [130, 131].

Chronic treatment with *L. rhamnosus* (JB-1) in mice lowered stress-induced corticosterone as well as anxiety- and depression-related behavior and caused alterations in Gamma-Aminobutyric acid [GABA(B1b) and GABA(Aα2)] receptor mRNA in specific regions within the brain [132]. Interestingly, these findings were not found in vagotomized mice [132]. The vagus is known to mediate communication between the gut microbiota and the HPA axis, with increased CRF mRNA, plasma ACTH, and corticosterone concentrations in rodents following vagal stimulation [133]. Furthermore, in humans, vagal nerve stimulation has antidepressant effects, including normalization of the HPA axis [134, 135]. In mice, JB-1 increased the firing rate of the mesenteric nerve bundle, which was prevented by subdiaphragmatic vagotomy [133]. Similarly, in a mouse model in which chronic mild DSS colitis induces anxiety-like behavior, *B. longum* NCC3001 normalized the anxiety-like behavior and CNS changes induced by chronic gut inflammation but not in mice that had undergone vagotomy [136]. Similar results were obtained in a *T. muris* parasite model of chronic colonic infection, further supporting a neurally mediated mechanism of the probiotic effect [103].

From an immunological perspective, Smith et al. demonstrated that *Recombination activating gene-1* (*Rag1*) knockout mice, which are B and T cell deficient, had a dysbiosis, altered behavior, and heightened HPA axis activity [137]. When pretreatment with *L. rhamnosus* (R0011) and L. *helveticus* (R0052) was administered, the microbiota and behavioral changes were normalized [137]. In rats, myocardial infarction (MI) is accompanied by increased cellular apoptosis in the limbic system and a depression-like behavior [138]. In this model, administration of probiotics that combined *L. helveticus*and *B. longum* ameliorated post-MI depression through reduction in pro-inflammatory cytokines and restoration of barrier integrity in the GI tract [139]. Interestingly, using the IL-10 knockout mouse, which is a model of colonic inflammation similar to IBD, Ohland et al. showed that the ingested diet and the presence or absence of inflammation within the GI tract can influence probiotic efficacy [140]. This suggests a role for immune cells in the intestinal and behavioral health in rodents. Collectively, these studies overwhelmingly support a role for probiotic strains in modulating various aspects of brain function and behavior, some of which appear to be at least partly vagal dependent.

4.1.2. Prebiotics

Prebiotics are food components that modulate the microbiota by enhancing the growth of probiotic microbes and have been used in several studies to further define a role for the microbiome in behavior. Human milk oligosaccharides (HMO) promote the growth of specific bacteria including probiotic members of the genus *Bifidobacterium* and *Lactobacillus*. Mice fed the prebiotic containing the human milk oligosaccharides 3′Sialyllactose (3′SL) or 6′Sialyllactose (6′SL) showed less anxiety-like behavior, and less microbiota alteration in response to stress [141]. The prebiotics, fructo-oligosaccharide (FOS), and galacto-oligosaccharides (GOS) promoted the growth of the *Lactobacilli* and *Bifidobacteria* in the gut and raised hippocampal BDNF and NR1 subunit expression compared with controls. GOS also increases hippocampal NR2A subunits and NR1 expression within the frontal cortex and increases plasma D-alanine, which acts as an agonist at the NMDA receptor [142]. These studies show that prebiotic-mediated proliferation of gut microbiota, like probiotics, can affect brain neurochemistry and animal behavior.

4.1.3. Antimicrobials

Administration of oral, but not intraperitoneal, antimicrobials (neomycin, bacitracin, and pimaricin) to SPF mice increased the proportion of *Lactobacilli* and *Actinobacteria* populations, while decreasing the proportion of *γ-proteobacteria* and *Bacteroidetes* populations [113]. These microbiota changes were associated with improvements in standardized tests of less apprehensive behavior, effects that were reversible after discontinuation of antimicrobial treatment and return to pretreatment microbiota profiles. These changes were independent of inflammation, levels of gastrointestinal neurotransmitters, and nervous system integrity.

4.2. Evidence from human studies

4.2.1. Microbial diversity among different populations

Cross-sectional studies in humans have begun to investigate the gut microbial composition and its association with mood. Naseribafrouei et al. analyzed fecal samples from patients with depression and controls and found no overall significant difference in species diversity between depressed and non-depressed samples but rather a general overrepresentation of the order *Bacteroidales* in depression and a decrease in family *Lachnospiraceae* [143]. At a genus level, *Alistipes* and *Oscillibacter* were associated with depression. Jiang et al. analyzed fecal samples from patients with active major depressive disorder (active-MDD), responded major depressive disorder (responded-MDD) and healthy controls. In contrast to the first study, Jiang et al. found increased fecal bacterial α-diversity in the active-MDD group when compared with controls; however, this was not found between the responded-MDD when compared with controls [144]. The three dominant phyla *Bacteroidetes, Proteobacteria,* and *Actinobacteria* were increased, while *Firmicutes* were significantly reduced in both active-MDD and responded-MDD groups than in controls. *Faecalibacterium* was associated with a negative correlation with the severity of depressive symptoms. Concordant with Naseribafrouei et al., an increase in *Oscillibacter* and *Alistipes* was found in depression compared to controls [144]. Of note, possible confounding elements to explain the differences between these two studies may be related to the recruitment of controls from an outpatient neurology clinic by Naseribafrouei et al., unlike Jiang who recruited healthy subjects as controls [143, 144]. Additionally, differences between ages of subjects as well as geographic locations between the studies could contribute to differences in bacterial diversity, as diversity of gut bacteria is known to be influenced by several factors including health status, age, diet, and antibiotic use [47]. In a cross-sectional observational study examining associations between the gut microbiome and maternally rated temperament in toddlers, it was found that certain dimensions of temperament could be associated with differences in phylogenetic diversity [145]. In addition, they found certain sex-specific associations between temperament and the gut microbiome.

These studies begin to identify bacterial groups potentially harmful in the pathogenesis of mood disorders, though further studies will be needed to elucidate temporal and causal relationships between gut microbiota and depression as well as to evaluate their utility as biomarkers of disease. Again, as in the rodent studies, these results point to sex-related differences in how the microbiome may be regulated and how it affects the CNS and behavior.

4.2.2. Human probiotic studies

To date, few probiotic studies have been conducted in humans to evaluate their effects on mood. The consumption of a 3-week course of a yogurt containing *Lactobacillus casei* Shirota (LcS) improved mood in patients with low mood (as evaluated by a questionnaire-based assessment) [146]. In healthy volunteers who received a 30-day course of *L. helveticus* R0052 and *B. longum* R0175 compared to placebo, probiotic-treated subjects displayed lower somatization, depression, and anger hostility [147]. A study by Steenbergen et al. aimed to complement these findings and showed that participants who received a multispecies probiotic had reduced cognitive reactivity to sad mood [148]. In a randomized double-blind placebo trial with chronic fatigue syndrome (CFS) patients, two months of daily LcS induced a significant rise in both *Lactobacillus* and *Bifidobacterium* and a concomitant significant decrease in anxiety symptoms compared to controls [149]. These results provide evidence that the intake of probiotics may help reduce negative thoughts associated with sad mood. Probiotic supplementation warrants further research as a potential treatment or preventative strategy for depression.

5. Perspectives

The topics discussed in this review emphasize the broad influence that the microbiome has in a wide range of psychiatric and neurologic diseases. Changes in the microbiome are relevant to many brain diseases and understanding what the abnormal changes in the GI microflora are in these conditions is necessary to identify novel targets for therapies. Recognition of pathological changes in the constitution of the microbiome offers a possible means of anticipating or prognosticating future disease. It also provides an opportunity to intervene and correct a dysbiosis with beneficial effects on the disease.

The role of the microbiome in neurodevelopment cannot be underestimated. As previously discussed, exposure to particular microorganisms at specific time points in animal models can have lasting impacts on neurological disease risk and behavior. Treatments that alter the microbial flora may influence healthy brain development and further work in this area is needed to appreciate how significant this may be in humans.

Future work that expands on our current understanding of the dysbioses that occur in CNS diseases should hopefully provide further insight into microbiota-related disease mechanisms and provide additional therapeutic options for patients.

Acknowledgements

This chapter was supported in part by the Department of Pathology, New York University Langone Medical Center, National Cancer Institute, National Institute of Allergy and Infectious Diseases, and National Institute of Dental and Craniofacial Research of the National

Institutes of Health under award numbers UH3CA140233, U01CA182370, R01CA159036, R01AI110372, and R21DE025352. ZP is a Staff Physician at the Department of Veterans Affairs New York Harbor Healthcare System. The content is solely the responsibility of the authors and does not necessarily represent the official views of the National Institutes of Health, the U.S. Department of Veterans Affairs, or the United States Government.

Dr. Hickman and Dr. Hussein equally contributed to this work.

Author details

Richard A. Hickman[1], Maryem A. Hussein[1] and Zhiheng Pei[1,2*]

*Address all correspondence to: zhiheng.pei@nyumc.org

1 New York University School of Medicine, New York, USA

2 Department of Veterans Affairs New York Harbor Healthcare System, New York, USA

References

[1] Gill SR, Pop M, Deboy RT, Eckburg PB, Turnbaugh PJ, Samuel BS, et al. Metagenomic analysis of the human distal gut microbiome. Science (New York, NY). 2006;312(5778): 1355–9.

[2] Lee WJ, Hase K. Gut microbiota-generated metabolites in animal health and disease. Nature Chemical Biology. 2014;10(6):416–24.

[3] Walker AW, Lawley TD. Therapeutic modulation of intestinal dysbiosis. Pharmacological Research. 2013;69(1):75–86.

[4] Forsythe P, Bienenstock J, Kunze WA. Vagal pathways for microbiome-brain-gut axis communication. Advances in Experimental Medicine and Biology. 2014;817:115–33.

[5] Simren M, Barbara G, Flint HJ, Spiegel BM, Spiller RC, Vanner S, et al. Intestinal microbiota in functional bowel disorders: A Rome foundation report. Gut. 2013;62(1): 159–76.

[6] Mayer EA, Savidge T, Shulman RJ. Brain-gut microbiome interactions and functional bowel disorders. Gastroenterology. 2014;146(6):1500–12.

[7] Konturek PC, Haziri D, Brzozowski T, Hess T, Heyman S, Kwiecien S, et al. Emerging role of fecal microbiota therapy in the treatment of gastrointestinal and extra-gastrointestinal diseases. Journal of Physiology and Pharmacology: An Official Journal of the Polish Physiological Society. 2015;66(4):483–91.

[8] Dominguez-Bello MG, Costello EK, Contreras M, Magris M, Hidalgo G, Fierer N, et al. Delivery mode shapes the acquisition and structure of the initial microbiota across multiple body habitats in newborns. Proceedings of the National Academy of Sciences of the United States of America. 2010;107(26):11971–5.

[9] Penders J, Thijs C, Vink C, Stelma FF, Snijders B, Kummeling I, et al. Factors influencing the composition of the intestinal microbiota in early infancy. Pediatrics. 2006;118(2): 511–21.

[10] Jimenez E, Marin ML, Martin R, Odriozola JM, Olivares M, Xaus J, et al. Is meconium from healthy newborns actually sterile? Research in Microbiology. 2008;159(3):187–93.

[11] Hansen R, Scott KP, Khan S, Martin JC, Berry SH, Stevenson M, et al. First-pass meconium samples from healthy term vaginally-delivered neonates: An analysis of the microbiota. PLoS One. 2015;10(7):e0133320.

[12] Borre YE, O'Keeffe GW, Clarke G, Stanton C, Dinan TG, Cryan JF. Microbiota and neurodevelopmental windows: Implications for brain disorders. Trends in Molecular Medicine. 2014;20(9):509–18.

[13] Diamond B, Huerta PT, Tracey K, Volpe BT. It takes guts to grow a brain: Increasing evidence of the important role of the intestinal microflora in neuro- and immune-modulatory functions during development and adulthood. Bioessays. 2011;33(8):588–91.

[14] Qin N, Yang F, Li A, Prifti E, Chen Y, Shao L, et al. Alterations of the human gut microbiome in liver cirrhosis. Nature. 2014;513(7516):59–64.

[15] Rai R, Saraswat VA, Dhiman RK. Gut microbiota: Its role in hepatic encephalopathy. Journal of Clinical and Experimental Hepatology. 2015;5(Suppl. 1):S29–36.

[16] Al Sibae MR, McGuire BM. Current trends in the treatment of hepatic encephalopathy. Therapeutics and Clinical Risk Management. 2009;5(3):617–26.

[17] Bajaj JS. Review article: Potential mechanisms of action of rifaximin in the management of hepatic encephalopathy and other complications of cirrhosis. Alimentary Pharmacology &Therapeutics. 2016;43(Suppl. 1):11–26.

[18] Haussinger D, Schliess F. Pathogenetic mechanisms of hepatic encephalopathy. Gut. 2008;57(8):1156–65.

[19] Ponziani FR, Gerardi V, Pecere S, D'Aversa F, Lopetuso L, Zocco MA, et al. Effect of rifaximin on gut microbiota composition in advanced liver disease and its complications. World Journal of Gastroenterology. 2015;21(43):12322–33.

[20] Bass NM, Mullen KD, Sanyal A, Poordad F, Neff G, Leevy CB, et al. Rifaximin treatment in hepatic encephalopathy. The New England Journal of Medicine. 2010;362(12):1071–81.

[21] Bajaj JS, Heuman DM, Sanyal AJ, Hylemon PB, Sterling RK, Stravitz RT, et al. Modulation of the metabiome by rifaximin in patients with cirrhosis and minimal hepatic encephalopathy. PLoS One. 2013;8(4):e60042.

[22] Lassmann H, Bruck W, Lucchinetti CF. The immunopathology of multiple sclerosis: An overview. Brain Pathology (Zurich, Switzerland). 2007;17(2):210–8.

[23] Lassmann H, van Horssen J, Mahad D. Progressive multiple sclerosis: Pathology and pathogenesis. Nature Reviews Neurology. 2012;8(11):647–56.

[24] Popescu BF, Lucchinetti CF. Pathology of demyelinating diseases. Annual Review of Pathology. 2012;7:185–217.

[25] Frohman EM, Racke MK, Raine CS. Multiple sclerosis – the plaque and its pathogenesis. The New England Journal of Medicine. 2006;354(9):942–55.

[26] Henderson AP, Barnett MH, Parratt JD, Prineas JW. Multiple sclerosis: Distribution of inflammatory cells in newly forming lesions. Annals of Neurology. 2009;66(6):739–53.

[27] Disanto G, Berlanga AJ, Handel AE, Para AE, Burrell AM, Fries A, et al. Heterogeneity in multiple sclerosis: Scratching the surface of a complex disease. Autoimmune Diseases. 2010;2011:932351.

[28] Compston A, Coles A. Multiple sclerosis. Lancet (London, England). 2008;372(9648): 1502–17.

[29] Bashinskaya VV, Kulakova OG, Boyko AN, Favorov AV, Favorova OO. A review of genome-wide association studies for multiple sclerosis: Classical and hypothesis-driven approaches. Human Genetics. 2015;134(11–12):1143–62.

[30] Compston A, Coles A. Multiple sclerosis. Lancet (London, England). 2002;359(9313): 1221–31.

[31] Simpson S, Jr., Blizzard L, Otahal P, Van der Mei I, Taylor B. Latitude is significantly associated with the prevalence of multiple sclerosis: A meta-analysis. Journal of Neurology, Neurosurgery, and Psychiatry. 2011;82(10):1132–41.

[32] Acheson ED, Bachrach CA, Wright FM. Some comments on the relationship of the distribution of multiple sclerosis to latitude, solar radiation, and other variables. Acta Psychiatrica Scandinavica Supplementum. 1960;35(147):132–47.

[33] Dean G, Kurtzke JF. On the risk of multiple sclerosis according to age at immigration to South Africa. British Medical Journal. 1971;3(5777):725–9.

[34] Yatsunenko T, Rey FE, Manary MJ, Trehan I, Dominguez-Bello MG, Contreras M, et al. Human gut microbiome viewed across age and geography. Nature. 2012;486(7402):222–7.

[35] Conlon MA, Bird AR. The impact of diet and lifestyle on gut microbiota and human health. Nutrients. 2015;7(1):17–44.

[36] Leibowitz U, Antonovsky A, Medalie JM, Smith HA, Halpern L, Alter M. Epidemiological study of multiple sclerosis in Israel. II. Multiple sclerosis and level of sanitation. Journal of Neurology, Neurosurgery, and Psychiatry. 1966;29(1):60–8.

[37] Strachan DP. Hay fever, hygiene, and household size. BMJ (Clinical research ed). 1989;299(6710):1259–60.

[38] Fleming J, Fabry Z. The hygiene hypothesis and multiple sclerosis. Annals of Neurology. 2007;61(2):85–9.

[39] Kurtzke JF, Heltberg A. Multiple sclerosis in the Faroe Islands: An epitome. Journal of Clinical Epidemiology. 2001;54(1):1–22.

[40] Kurtzke JF, Hyllested K. MS epidemiology in Faroe Islands. Rivista di Neurologia. 1987;57(2):77–87.

[41] Wallin MT, Heltberg A, Kurtzke JF. Multiple sclerosis in the Faroe Islands. 8. Notifiable diseases. Acta Neurologica Scandinavica. 2010;122(2):102–9.

[42] Hawkes CH. Smoking is a risk factor for multiple sclerosis: A metanalysis. Multiple Sclerosis (Houndmills, Basingstoke, England). 2007;13(5):610–5.

[43] Hernan MA, Olek MJ, Ascherio A. Cigarette smoking and incidence of multiple sclerosis. American Journal of Epidemiology. 2001;154(1):69–74.

[44] Alonso A, Hernan MA. Temporal trends in the incidence of multiple sclerosis: A systematic review. Neurology. 2008;71(2):129–35.

[45] Kampman MT, Brustad M. Vitamin D: A candidate for the environmental effect in multiple sclerosis – observations from Norway. Neuroepidemiology. 2008;30(3):140–6.

[46] Munger KL, Chitnis T, Ascherio A. Body size and risk of MS in two cohorts of US women. Neurology. 2009;73(19):1543–50.

[47] Dominianni C, Sinha R, Goedert JJ, Pei Z, Yang L, Hayes RB, et al. Sex, body mass index, and dietary fiber intake influence the human gut microbiome. PLoS One. 2015;10(4):e0124599.

[48] Tankou S, Bry L, Gerber G, Lin N, Glanz B, Cook S, et al. Effect of Vitamin D level in the gut microbiome of MS patients (P2.206). Neurology. 2015;84(14 Suppl.).

[49] Mielcarz DW, Kasper LH. The gut microbiome in multiple sclerosis. Current Treatment Options in Neurology. 2015;17(4):344.

[50] Sriram S, Steiner I. Experimental allergic encephalomyelitis: A misleading model of multiple sclerosis. Annals of Neurology. 2005;58(6):939–45.

[51] Lassmann H. Experimental models of multiple sclerosis. Revue Neurologique. 2007;163(6–7):651–5.

[52] Falk PG, Hooper LV, Midtvedt T, Gordon JI. Creating and maintaining the gastrointestinal ecosystem: What we know and need to know from gnotobiology. Microbiology and Molecular Biology Reviews. 1998;62(4):1157–70.

[53] Bauer H, Horowitz RE, Levenson SM, Popper H. The response of the lymphatic tissue to the microbial flora. Studies on germfree mice. The American Journal of Pathology. 1963;42:471–83.

[54] Chervonsky AV. Influence of microbial environment on autoimmunity. Nature Immunology. 2010;11(1):28–35.

[55] Berer K, Mues M, Koutrolos M, Rasbi ZA, Boziki M, Johner C, et al. Commensal microbiota and myelin autoantigen cooperate to trigger autoimmune demyelination. Nature. 2011;479(7374):538–41.

[56] Lee YK, Menezes JS, Umesaki Y, Mazmanian SK. Proinflammatory T-cell responses to gut microbiota promote experimental autoimmune encephalomyelitis. Proceedings of the National Academy of Sciences of the United States of America. 2011;108(Suppl. 1): 4615–22.

[57] Ivanov, II, Atarashi K, Manel N, Brodie EL, Shima T, Karaoz U, et al. Induction of intestinal Th17 cells by segmented filamentous bacteria. Cell. 2009;139(3):485–98.

[58] Miyake S, Kim S, Suda W, Oshima K, Nakamura M, Matsuoka T, et al. Dysbiosis in the gut microbiota of patients with multiple sclerosis, with a striking depletion of species belonging to clostridia XIVa and IV clusters. PLoS One. 2015;10(9):e0137429.

[59] Joossens M, Huys G, Cnockaert M, De Preter V, Verbeke K, Rutgeerts P, et al. Dysbiosis of the faecal microbiota in patients with Crohn's disease and their unaffected relatives. Gut. 2011;60(5):631–7.

[60] Rumah KR, Linden J, Fischetti VA, Vartanian T. Isolation of *Clostridium perfringens* type B in an individual at first clinical presentation of multiple sclerosis provides clues for environmental triggers of the disease. PLoS One. 2013;8(10):e76359.

[61] Linden JR, Ma Y, Zhao B, Harris JM, Rumah KR, Schaeren-Wiemers N, et al. Clostridium perfringens epsilon toxin causes selective death of mature oligodendrocytes and central nervous system demyelination. mBio. 2015;6(3):e02513.

[62] Wioland L, Dupont JL, Doussau F, Gaillard S, Heid F, Isope P, et al. Epsilon toxin from Clostridium perfringens acts on oligodendrocytes without forming pores, and causes demyelination. Cellular Microbiology. 2015;17(3):369–88.

[63] Jhangi S, Gandhi R, Glanz B, Cook S, Nejad P, Ward D, et al. Increased Archaea species and changes with therapy in gut microbiome of mutliple sclerosis subjects (S24.001). Neurology. 2014;82(10).

[64] Tremlett H, Fadrosh D, Lynch S, Hart J, Graves J, Lulu S, et al. Gut microbiome in early pediatric multiple sclerosis: A case-control study (P4.027). Neurology. 2015;84(14 Suppl.).

[65] Libbey JE, Cusick MF, Fujinami RS. Role of pathogens in multiple sclerosis. International Reviews of Immunology. 2014;33(4):266–83.

[66] Sixbey JW, Nedrud JG, Raab-Traub N, Hanes RA, Pagano JS. Epstein-Barr virus replication in oropharyngeal epithelial cells. The New England Journal of Medicine. 1984;310(19):1225–30.

[67] Haahr S, Hollsberg P. Multiple sclerosis is linked to Epstein-Barr virus infection. Reviews in Medical Virology. 2006;16(5):297–310.

[68] Belbasis L, Bellou V, Evangelou E, Ioannidis JP, Tzoulaki I. Environmental risk factors and multiple sclerosis: An umbrella review of systematic reviews and meta-analyses. The Lancet Neurology. 2015;14(3):263–73.

[69] Thacker EL, Mirzaei F, Ascherio A. Infectious mononucleosis and risk for multiple sclerosis: A meta-analysis. Annals of Neurology. 2006;59(3):499–503.

[70] Handel AE, Williamson AJ, Disanto G, Handunnetthi L, Giovannoni G, Ramagopalan SV. An updated meta-analysis of risk of multiple sclerosis following infectious mononucleosis. PLoS One. 2010;5(9).

[71] Serafini B, Rosicarelli B, Franciotta D, Magliozzi R, Reynolds R, Cinque P, et al. Dysregulated Epstein-Barr virus infection in the multiple sclerosis brain. The Journal of Experimental Medicine. 2007;204(12):2899–912.

[72] Colombo M, Dono M, Gazzola P, Roncella S, Valetto A, Chiorazzi N, et al. Accumulation of clonally related B lymphocytes in the cerebrospinal fluid of multiple sclerosis patients. Journal of Immunology (Baltimore, Md: 1950). 2000;164(5): 2782–9.

[73] Cepok S, Zhou D, Srivastava R, Nessler S, Stei S, Bussow K, et al. Identification of Epstein-Barr virus proteins as putative targets of the immune response in multiple sclerosis. The Journal of Clinical Investigation. 2005;115(5):1352–60.

[74] Correale J, Farez M. Association between parasite infection and immune responses in multiple sclerosis. Annals of Neurology. 2007;61(2):97–108.

[75] Correale J, Farez M, Razzitte G. Helminth infections associated with multiple sclerosis induce regulatory B cells. Annals of Neurology. 2008;64(2):187–99.

[76] Duddy M, Niino M, Adatia F, Hebert S, Freedman M, Atkins H, et al. Distinct effector cytokine profiles of memory and naive human B cell subsets and implication in multiple sclerosis. Journal of Immunology (Baltimore, Md: 1950). 2007;178(10):6092–9.

[77] Fleming JO, Isaak A, Lee JE, Luzzio CC, Carrithers MD, Cook TD, et al. Probiotic helminth administration in relapsing-remitting multiple sclerosis: A phase 1 study. Multiple Sclerosis (Houndmills, Basingstoke, England). 2011;17(6):743–54.

[78] Benzel F, Erdur H, Kohler S, Frentsch M, Thiel A, Harms L, et al. Immune monitoring of Trichuris suis egg therapy in multiple sclerosis patients. Journal of Helminthology. 2012;86(3):339–47.

[79] Postuma RB, Berg D, Stern M, Poewe W, Olanow CW, Oertel W, et al. MDS clinical diagnostic criteria for Parkinson's disease. Movement Disorders. 2015;30(12):1591–601.

[80] Gelb DJ, Oliver E, Gilman S. Diagnostic criteria for Parkinson disease. Archives of Neurology. 1999;56(1):33–9.

[81] Braak H, Del Tredici K, Rub U, de Vos RA, Jansen Steur EN, Braak E. Staging of brain pathology related to sporadic Parkinson's disease. Neurobiology of Aging. 2003;24(2): 197–211.

[82] Savica R, Carlin JM, Grossardt BR, Bower JH, Ahlskog JE, Maraganore DM, et al. Medical records documentation of constipation preceding Parkinson disease: A case-control study. Neurology. 2009;73(21):1752–8.

[83] Cersosimo MG, Raina GB, Pecci C, Pellene A, Calandra CR, Gutierrez C, et al. Gastrointestinal manifestations in Parkinson's disease: Prevalence and occurrence before motor symptoms. Journal of Neurology. 2013;260(5):1332–8.

[84] Sakakibara R, Odaka T, Uchiyama T, Asahina M, Yamaguchi K, Yamaguchi T, et al. Colonic transit time and rectoanal videomanometry in Parkinson's disease. Journal of Neurology, Neurosurgery, and Psychiatry. 2003;74(2):268–72.

[85] Wakabayashi K, Takahashi H, Takeda S, Ohama E, Ikuta F. Parkinson's disease: The presence of Lewy bodies in Auerbach's and Meissner's plexuses. Acta Neuropathologica. 1988;76(3):217–21.

[86] Wakabayashi K, Takahashi H, Takeda S, Ohama E, Ikuta F. Lewy bodies in the enteric nervous system in Parkinson's disease. Archives of Histology and Cytology. 1989;52(Suppl):191–4.

[87] Cersosimo MG, Perandones C, Micheli FE, Raina GB, Beron AM, Nasswetter G, et al. Alpha-synuclein immunoreactivity in minor salivary gland biopsies of Parkinson's disease patients. Movement Disorders. 2011;26(1):188–90.

[88] Abbott RD, Petrovitch H, White LR, Masaki KH, Tanner CM, Curb JD, et al. Frequency of bowel movements and the future risk of Parkinson's disease. Neurology. 2001;57(3): 456–62.

[89] Shannon KM, Keshavarzian A, Dodiya HB, Jakate S, Kordower JH. Is alpha-synuclein in the colon a biomarker for premotor Parkinson's disease? Evidence from 3 cases. Movement Disorders. 2012;27(6):716–9.

[90] Pan-Montojo F, Schwarz M, Winkler C, Arnhold M, O'Sullivan GA, Pal A, et al. Environmental toxins trigger PD-like progression via increased alpha-synuclein release from enteric neurons in mice. Scientific Reports. 2012;2:898.

[91] Li JY, Englund E, Holton JL, Soulet D, Hagell P, Lees AJ, et al. Lewy bodies in grafted neurons in subjects with Parkinson's disease suggest host-to-graft disease propagation. Nature Medicine. 2008;14(5):501–3.

[92] Kordower JH, Brundin P. Lewy body pathology in long-term fetal nigral transplants: Is Parkinson's disease transmitted from one neural system to another? Neuropsychopharmacology. 2009;34(1):254.

[93] Svensson E, Horvath-Puho E, Thomsen RW, Djurhuus JC, Pedersen L, Borghammer P, et al. Vagotomy and subsequent risk of Parkinson's disease. Annals of Neurology. 2015;78(4):522–9.

[94] Scheperjans F, Aho V, Pereira PA, Koskinen K, Paulin L, Pekkonen E, et al. Gut microbiota are related to Parkinson's disease and clinical phenotype. Movement Disorders. 2015;30(3):350–8.

[95] Tan AH, Mahadeva S, Thalha AM, Gibson PR, Kiew CK, Yeat CM, et al. Small intestinal bacterial overgrowth in Parkinson's disease. Parkinsonism & Related Disorders. 2014;20(5):535–40.

[96] Fasano A, Bove F, Gabrielli M, Petracca M, Zocco MA, Ragazzoni E, et al. The role of small intestinal bacterial overgrowth in Parkinson's disease. Movement Disorders. 2013;28(9):1241–9.

[97] Hubbard PS, Esiri MM, Reading M, McShane R, Nagy Z. Alpha-synuclein pathology in the olfactory pathways of dementia patients. Journal of Anatomy. 2007;211(1):117–24.

[98] Lydiard RB. Irritable bowel syndrome, anxiety, and depression: What are the links? The Journal of Clinical Psychiatry. 2001;62(Suppl. 8):38–45; discussion 6–7.

[99] Lydiard RB, Fossey MD, Marsh W, Ballenger JC. Prevalence of psychiatric disorders in patients with irritable bowel syndrome. Psychosomatics. 1993;34(3):229–34.

[100] Helzer JE, Chammas S, Norland CC, Stillings WA, Alpers DH. A study of the association between Crohn's disease and psychiatric illness. Gastroenterology. 1984;86(2):324–30.

[101] Helzer JE, Stillings WA, Chammas S, Norland CC, Alpers DH. A controlled study of the association between ulcerative colitis and psychiatric diagnoses. Digestive Diseases and Sciences. 1982;27(6):513–8.

[102] Andrews H, Barczak P, Allan RN. Psychiatric illness in patients with inflammatory bowel disease. Gut. 1987;28(12):1600–4.

[103] Bercik P, Verdu EF, Foster JA, Macri J, Potter M, Huang X, et al. Chronic gastrointestinal inflammation induces anxiety-like behavior and alters central nervous system biochemistry in mice. Gastroenterology. 2010;139(6):2102–12.e1.

[104] Tannock GW, Savage DC. Influences of dietary and environmental stress on microbial populations in the murine gastrointestinal tract. Infection and Immunity. 1974;9(3):591–8.

[105] Smith SM, Vale WW. The role of the hypothalamic-pituitary-adrenal axis in neuroendocrine responses to stress. Dialogues in Clinical Neuroscience. 2006;8(4):383–95.

[106] Merali Z, Du L, Hrdina P, Palkovits M, Faludi G, Poulter MO, et al. Dysregulation in the suicide brain: mRNA expression of corticotropin-releasing hormone receptors and GABA(A) receptor subunits in frontal cortical brain region. The Journal of Neuroscience: The Official Journal of the Society for Neuroscience. 2004;24(6):1478–85.

[107] Burke HM, Davis MC, Otte C, Mohr DC. Depression and cortisol responses to psychological stress: A meta-analysis. Psychoneuroendocrinology. 2005;30(9):846–56.

[108] Sudo N, Chida Y, Aiba Y, Sonoda J, Oyama N, Yu XN, et al. Postnatal microbial colonization programs the hypothalamic-pituitary-adrenal system for stress response in mice. The Journal of Physiology. 2004;558(Pt 1):263–75.

[109] Clarke G, Grenham S, Scully P, Fitzgerald P, Moloney RD, Shanahan F, et al. The microbiome-gut-brain axis during early life regulates the hippocampal serotonergic system in a sex-dependent manner. Molecular Psychiatry. 2013;18(6):666–73.

[110] Diaz Heijtz R, Wang S, Anuar F, Qian Y, Bjorkholm B, Samuelsson A, et al. Normal gut microbiota modulates brain development and behavior. Proceedings of the National Academy of Sciences of the United States of America. 2011;108(7):3047–52.

[111] Neufeld KM, Kang N, Bienenstock J, Foster JA. Reduced anxiety-like behavior and central neurochemical change in germ-free mice. Neurogastroenterology and Motility: The Official Journal of the European Gastrointestinal Motility Society. 2011;23(3):255–64, e119.

[112] Nishino R, Mikami K, Takahashi H, Tomonaga S, Furuse M, Hiramoto T, et al. Commensal microbiota modulate murine behaviors in a strictly contamination-free environment confirmed by culture-based methods. Neurogastroenterology and Motility: The Official Journal of the European Gastrointestinal Motility Society. 2013;25(6):521–8.

[113] Bercik P, Denou E, Collins J, Jackson W, Lu J, Jury J, et al. The intestinal microbiota affect central levels of brain-derived neurotropic factor and behavior in mice. Gastroenterology. 2011;141(2):599-609, e1–3.

[114] Delgado PL. Depression: The case for a monoamine deficiency. The Journal of Clinical Psychiatry. 2000;61(Suppl. 6):7–11.

[115] Mohler H. The GABA system in anxiety and depression and its therapeutic potential. Neuropharmacology. 2012;62(1):42–53.

[116] Mann JJ. Role of the serotonergic system in the pathogenesis of major depression and suicidal behavior. Neuropsychopharmacology. 1999;21(S1):99S–105S.

[117] Kahn RS, van Praag HM, Wetzler S, Asnis GM, Barr G. Serotonin and anxiety revisited. Biological Psychiatry. 1988;23(2):189–208.

[118] Bremner JD, Krystal JH, Southwick SM, Charney DS. Noradrenergic mechanisms in stress and anxiety: I. Preclinical studies. Synapse (New York, NY). 1996;23(1):28–38.

[119] Stein DJ, Westenberg HG, Liebowitz MR. Social anxiety disorder and generalized anxiety disorder: Serotonergic and dopaminergic neurocircuitry. The Journal of Clinical Psychiatry. 2002;63(Suppl. 6):12–9.

[120] Crumeyrolle-Arias M, Jaglin M, Bruneau A, Vancassel S, Cardona A, Dauge V, et al. Absence of the gut microbiota enhances anxiety-like behavior and neuroendocrine response to acute stress in rats. Psychoneuroendocrinology. 2014;42:207–17.

[121] Smith KA, Fairburn CG, Cowen PJ. Relapse of depression after rapid depletion of tryptophan. Lancet (London, England). 1997;349(9056):915–9.

[122] Cowen PJ, Parry-Billings M, Newsholme EA. Decreased plasma tryptophan levels in major depression. Journal of Affective Disorders. 1989;16(1):27–31.

[123] Capuron L, Ravaud A, Neveu PJ, Miller AH, Maes M, Dantzer R. Association between decreased serum tryptophan concentrations and depressive symptoms in cancer patients undergoing cytokine therapy. Molecular Psychiatry. 2002;7(5):468–73.

[124] Matsumoto M, Kibe R, Ooga T, Aiba Y, Sawaki E, Koga Y, et al. Cerebral low-molecular metabolites influenced by intestinal microbiota: A pilot study. Frontiers in Systems Neuroscience. 2013;7:9.

[125] Calabrese F, Rossetti AC, Racagni G, Gass P, Riva MA, Molteni R. Brain-derived neurotrophic factor: A bridge between inflammation and neuroplasticity. Frontiers in Cellular Neuroscience. 2014;8:430.

[126] Stilling RM, Ryan FJ, Hoban AE, Shanahan F, Clarke G, Claesson MJ, et al. Microbes & neurodevelopment – Absence of microbiota during early life increases activity-related transcriptional pathways in the amygdala. Brain, Behavior, and Immunity. 2015;50:209–20.

[127] Liang S, Wang T, Hu X, Luo J, Li W, Wu X, et al. Administration of Lactobacillus helveticus NS8 improves behavioral, cognitive, and biochemical aberrations caused by chronic restraint stress. Neuroscience. 2015;310:561–77.

[128] Ait-Belgnaoui A, Colom A, Braniste V, Ramalho L, Marrot A, Cartier C, et al. Probiotic gut effect prevents the chronic psychological stress-induced brain activity abnormality

in mice. Neurogastroenterology and Motility: The Official Journal of the European Gastrointestinal Motility Society. 2014;26(4):510–20.

[129] Savignac HM, Kiely B, Dinan TG, Cryan JF. Bifidobacteria exert strain-specific effects on stress-related behavior and physiology in BALB/c mice. Neurogastroenterology and Motility: The Official Journal of the European Gastrointestinal Motility Society. 2014;26(11):1615–27.

[130] Desbonnet L, Garrett L, Clarke G, Bienenstock J, Dinan TG. The probiotic Bifidobacteria infantis: An assessment of potential antidepressant properties in the rat. Journal of Psychiatric Research. 2008;43(2):164–74.

[131] Desbonnet L, Garrett L, Clarke G, Kiely B, Cryan JF, Dinan TG. Effects of the probiotic Bifidobacterium infantis in the maternal separation model of depression. Neuroscience. 2010;170(4):1179–88.

[132] Bravo JA, Forsythe P, Chew MV, Escaravage E, Savignac HM, Dinan TG, et al. Ingestion of Lactobacillus strain regulates emotional behavior and central GABA receptor expression in a mouse via the vagus nerve. Proceedings of National Academy of Sciencesof the United States of America. 2011;108(38):16050–5.

[133] Perez-Burgos A, Wang B, Mao YK, Mistry B, McVey Neufeld KA, Bienenstock J, et al. Psychoactive bacteria Lactobacillus rhamnosus (JB-1) elicits rapid frequency facilitation in vagal afferents. American Journal of Physiology Gastrointestinal and Liver Physiology. 2013;304(2):G211–20.

[134] Nemeroff CB, Mayberg HS, Krahl SE, McNamara J, Frazer A, Henry TR, et al. VNS therapy in treatment-resistant depression: Clinical evidence and putative neurobiological mechanisms. Neuropsychopharmacology. 2006;31(7):1345–55.

[135] O'Keane V, Dinan TG, Scott L, Corcoran C. Changes in hypothalamic-pituitary-adrenal axis measures after vagus nerve stimulation therapy in chronic depression. Biological Psychiatry. 2005;58(12):963–8.

[136] Bercik P, Park AJ, Sinclair D, Khoshdel A, Lu J, Huang X, et al. The anxiolytic effect of Bifidobacterium longum NCC3001 involves vagal pathways for gut-brain communication. Neurogastroenterology and Motility. 2011;23(12):1132–9.

[137] Smith CJ, Emge JR, Berzins K, Lung L, Khamishon R, Shah P, et al. Probiotics normalize the gut-brain-microbiota axis in immunodeficient mice. American Journal of Physiology Gastrointestinal and Liver Physiology. 2014;307(8):G793–802.

[138] Wann BP, Bah TM, Boucher M, Courtemanche J, Le Marec N, Rousseau G, et al. Vulnerability for apoptosis in the limbic system after myocardial infarction in rats: A possible model for human postinfarct major depression. Journal of Psychiatry & Neuroscience. 2007;32(1):11–6.

[139] Arseneault-Breard J, Rondeau I, Gilbert K, Girard SA, Tompkins TA, Godbout R, et al. Combination of Lactobacillus helveticus R0052 and Bifidobacterium longum R0175

reduces post-myocardial infarction depression symptoms and restores intestinal permeability in a rat model. The British Journal of Nutrition. 2012;107(12):1793–9.

[140] Ohland CL, Kish L, Bell H, Thiesen A, Hotte N, Pankiv E, et al. Effects of Lactobacillus helveticus on murine behavior are dependent on diet and genotype and correlate with alterations in the gut microbiome. Psychoneuroendocrinology. 2013;38(9):1738–47.

[141] Tarr AJ, Galley JD, Fisher SE, Chichlowski M, Berg BM, Bailey MT. The prebiotics 3'Sialyllactose and 6'Sialyllactose diminish stressor-induced anxiety-like behavior and colonic microbiota alterations: Evidence for effects on the gut-brain axis. Brain, Behavior, and Immunity. 2015;50:166–77.

[142] Savignac HM, Corona G, Mills H, Chen L, Spencer JP, Tzortzis G, et al. Prebiotic feeding elevates central brain derived neurotrophic factor, N-methyl-D-aspartate receptor subunits and D-serine. Neurochemistry International. 2013;63(8):756–64.

[143] Naseribafrouei A, Hestad K, Avershina E, Sekelja M, Linlokken A, Wilson R, et al. Correlation between the human fecal microbiota and depression. Neurogastroenterology and Motility: The Official Journal of the European Gastrointestinal Motility Society. 2014;26(8):1155–62.

[144] Jiang H, Ling Z, Zhang Y, Mao H, Ma Z, Yin Y, et al. Altered fecal microbiota composition in patients with major depressive disorder. Brain, Behavior, and Immunity. 2015;48:186–94.

[145] Christian LM, Galley JD, Hade EM, Schoppe-Sullivan S, Kamp Dush C, Bailey MT. Gut microbiome composition is associated with temperament during early childhood. Brain, Behavior, and Immunity. 2015;45:118–27.

[146] Benton D, Williams C, Brown A. Impact of consuming a milk drink containing a probiotic on mood and cognition. European Journal of Clinical Nutrition. 2007;61(3): 355–61.

[147] Messaoudi M, Violle N, Bisson JF, Desor D, Javelot H, Rougeot C. Beneficial psychological effects of a probiotic formulation (Lactobacillus helveticus R0052 and Bifidobacterium longum R0175) in healthy human volunteers. Gut Microbes. 2011;2(4):256–61.

[148] Steenbergen L, Sellaro R, van Hemert S, Bosch JA, Colzato LS. A randomized controlled trial to test the effect of multispecies probiotics on cognitive reactivity to sad mood. Brain, Behavior, and Immunity. 2015;48:258–64.

[149] Rao AV, Bested AC, Beaulne TM, Katzman MA, Iorio C, Berardi JM, et al. A randomized, double-blind, placebo-controlled pilot study of a probiotic in emotional symptoms of chronic fatigue syndrome. Gut Pathogens. 2009;1(1):6.

Section 4

Cardiovascular Disease and Gut Microbiota

Chapter 4

Role of Gut Microbiota in Cardiovascular Disease that Links to Host Genotype and Diet

Hein Min Tun, Frederick C. Leung and
Kimberly M. Cheng

Additional information is available at the end of the chapter

http://dx.doi.org/10.5772/64636

Abstract

Cardiovascular diseases (CVDs) are major outcomes of metabolic impairments in humans, which result from several genetic and environmental factors. In recent years, a 'microbiome hypothesis' has been proposed as a result of several studies that have attempted to understand underlying mechanisms of CVDs. Similar to CVDs, both genetic and environmental factors, especially diets, have a major impact on shaping gut microbiota and their functions. In the past decade, strong evidence has emerged to confirm the role of gut microbiota in contributing to the onset of CVDs. However, a comprehensive understanding of interactions among diet, host genotype, gut microbiota and CVDs is still facing challenges due to the complicated nature of CVDs. In this chapter, we review the present state of our knowledge about the contributory role of gut microbiota in CVDs and discuss the knowledge gaps that warrant further investigations. Moreover, we review the potential intervention strategies that may target the microbiota-driven pathology in CVDs and discuss the strength and weakness of animal models in studying the roles of gut microbiota in CVDs.

Keywords: gut microbiome, cardiovascular disease, host genotype, diet

1. Introduction

Cardiovascular disease (CVD) is a leading cause of death in industrialized societies, with increasing incidence in developing countries [1]. A combination of genetic and environmental factors contributes to risk for developing CVD [2]. A significant portion of CVDs can be attributed to ischemic heart disease, often a result of underlying coronary arterial diseases

INTECH
open science | open minds

© 2016 The Author(s). Licensee InTech. This chapter is distributed under the terms of the Creative Commons Attribution License (http://creativecommons.org/licenses/by/3.0), which permits unrestricted use, distribution, and reproduction in any medium, provided the original work is properly cited.

such as atherosclerosis. Risk factors for atherosclerosis include dyslipidaemia, hypertension, obesity, smoking, and diabetes [3, 4]. Extensive searching in recent years for causal genetic variants found less than one-fifth of CVD risk is accounted for by genetic determinants [5, 6]. Excluding tobacco exposure, dietary intake is our largest environmental risk, as we consume kilogram quantities into our bodies daily. However, specific dietary composition and precise quantification of dietary intake of a given individual are often difficult to assess.

Over the past decade, there has been a growing body of knowledge on the ecological diversity of microbes living symbiotically within us, especially in our gastrointestinal tract. More than 100 trillion microbial cells reside in the human gut, which is far outnumbering the host cells of the human body [7]. Microbial symbionts in our gastrointestinal system have coevolved with us and critically contribute to a variety of physiologic and metabolic processes of our body. Undeniably, human DNA is estimated to represent less than one-tenth of the total DNA within our bodies due to the remarkably large number of microorganisms in and on us, mainly within our gastrointestinal tract [8]. The composition of the microbial community in our gut can be largely affected not only by dietary exposures but also by genetic variants of the host, as well as any changes that impaired host's physiology and homeostasis. In recent years, although there is increasing evidence supporting an association between gut microbiota and diseases in human and animals [9, 10], the participatory roles of gut microbiota in our health, immune function, and disease initiation and progression have just begun to be explored. There has been an established understating of the role of microbial dysbiosis in the pathogenesis of some diseases of altered intestinal health [11]. The alteration of gut microbiota may contribute enormously to the digestion of food and absorption of metabolites, which further contribute to the development of a range of CVDs from atherosclerosis to cardiorenal dysfunction [12].

The gastrointestinal ecosystem is arguably the largest endocrine as well as paracrine organ in the body, producing a variety of biologically active compounds that may be transported in the systemic circulation and distributed to other organ systems within the host, thereby influencing diverse essential biochemical processes [12]. This chapter summarizes recent developments in our knowledge of the contributory role of gut microbiota on the initial onset and development of CVDs, and how diets and genetics of the host participate in their development. Potential strategies that can modulate gut microbiota for prevention and therapeutic interventions for CVDs will also be discussed.

2. Intestinal microbiota in cardiovascular disease—the good, the bad, and the ugly

The understanding of the link between gut microbiota and CVD was limited until the late 1990s. The fact that axenic (germ-free) ApoE knockout mice were not protected from the development of atherosclerosis suggested that the gut microbiota is not important in the pathogenesis of atherosclerosis [13]. A meta-analysis of clinical trials revealed that the modification of gut microbiota by antibiotics failed to demonstrate any benefit with regard to mortality due to cardiovascular events in coronary artery disease patients [14]. Furthermore, in an extensive study involving 4012 patients with stable coronary artery disease, the administration of azithromycin showed no effect on the risk of cardiac events [15]. However, the composition of the microbiota was shown to increase the severity of myocardial infarction in a Dahl S rat model of ischaemia/reperfusion injury of the heart, in which the authors indicated that vancomycin, a poorly absorbable antibiotic, reduced 27% of myocardial infarctions and increased 35% postischaemic mechanical function recovery [16]. This effect was associated with a change in the gut microbiota (both bacteria and fungi) and a reduction of plasma leptin, which was later confirmed by administration of the leptin-suppressing probiotic *Lactobacillus plantarum* 299v [16]. These earliest contradictory findings of antibiotic utilization (azithromycin vs. vancomycin) explained the complexity of gut microbiota-based intervention in terms of efficacy and properties of the applied protocol.

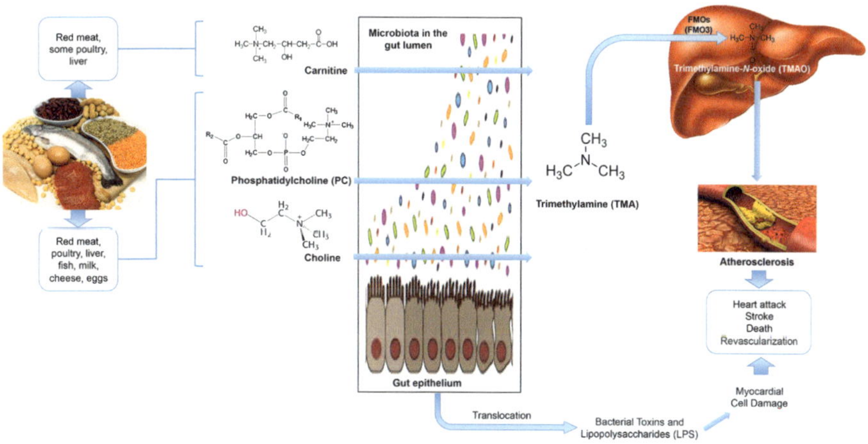

Figure 1. Gut microbiota and its impacts on atherosclerosis and major cardiovascular events through both nutrient/meta-organismal pathways that contribute TMAO formation and translocation of bacterial toxins that cause myocardial cell damage.

Invasion of indigenous and/or pathogenic oral and intestinal bacteria, as well as their metabolites and toxins into the vascular system, has been demonstrated in association with several CVD events [17, 18], although a causal association between periodontal infection and atherosclerotic CVD or its sequel has not been demonstrated. Periodontitis, also known as periodontal disease (PD), is an inflammatory disease of the oral cavity due to chronic bacterial infection of soft and hard tissues of the gum, mainly by Gram-negative bacteria [19]. A high-fat diet can induce not only metabolic alteration but also increased systolic and diastolic pressure in diabetic mice after longer term colonization with periodontal pathogens, such as *Porphyromonas gingivalis*, *Prevotella intermedia*, and *Fusobacterium nucleatum* [20]. The molecular mechanisms underlying this pathogenic phenotype is linked to bacterial lipopolysaccharide (LPS), which may increase oxidative stress and mitochondrial dysfunction that are responsible for inflammation-induced CVD (**Figure 1**) [21]. Endotoxin levels were shown to be higher in the hepatic veins compared with the left ventricle (LV) or pulmonary artery, suggesting possible endotoxin translocation from the gut into the circulation [22].

In recent years, more studies have highlighted the contributory role of gut microbiota in CVD. Initial hypothesis-generating studies using untargeted metabolomics analyses of plasma samples identified three metabolites, including phosphatidylcholine (PC; lecithin) metabolism-choline, betaine, and trimethylamine-N-oxide (TMAO) that are potentially associated with cardiovascular risk [23]. Another study also found increased concentration of the metabolite TMAO in patients with atherosclerosis and their correlation with this pathology [24]. Gut microbiota has been demonstrated to be responsible for TMAO synthesis by converting choline, an essential nutrient, into TMA. Subsequent oxidation of TMA through flavin monooxygenase 3 (FMO3) from the liver formed TMAO [25–27]. As an example, the bacteria belonging to *Erysipelotrichia* under the phylum Firmicutes can metabolize choline to TMA [24]. TMA is subsequently absorbed and rapidly oxidized by hepatic cells to form TMAO [28], which is responsible for macrophage foam cell formation by reducing reverse cholesterol transport and consequently promoting cholesterol accumulation in the foam cells of atheroma (**Figure 1**) [29]. However, the molecular mechanisms by which TMAO reduces reverse cholesterol transport are not well understood. These bacteria probably promote not only atherosclerosis through TMA-TMAO production but also non-alcoholic fatty live disease (NAFLD) by reducing choline availability for the synthesis of very low-density lipoprotein in the liver, resulting in triglyceride accumulation in the hepatocytes [30]. Furthermore, the abundance of such bacteria is also associated with an iron-rich diet. Such a diet promotes gut epithelial cell stress through iron accumulation in the enterocytes and consequently inflammation-induced dysbiosis of the gut microbiota in favour of *Erysipelotrichia* bacteria. Thus, an iron-rich diet may promote the development of NAFLD and atherosclerosis through alteration of the gut microbiota [31]. The dysbiosis of gut microbiota has been found in several metabolic diseases, including CVD. However, in different situations, dysbiosis can either be a cause or an effect of the disease or a spiralling cycle. In the case of CVDs, the dysbiosis of gut microbiota needs further investigation to determine whether it is cause or effect or both. Beside TMAO, intestinal bacteria produce certain toxins, such as indoxyl sulphate, p-cresyl sulphate, amines, and ammonia, which can later be eliminated by the kidneys in healthy individuals. In chronic kidney disease patients, however, these toxins may accumulate in the body of the patients.

In addition to the three bacterial metabolites described previously, L-carnitine has also been shown to accelerate atherosclerosis in mouse models, but only in the presence of intact gut microbiota and TMA/TMAO generation. High carnitine levels significantly increased the risk of myocardial infarction (MI), stroke, or death in experimental subjects with concurrently high TMAO levels. Similar to PC/choline, L-carnitine is a TMA-containing compound that releases TMA through the gut microbiota and consequently converted into TMAO by hepatic FMO (**Figure 1**) [29]. Thus, intestinal microbiota may play an obligatory role in generating TMAO from multiple dietary nutrients, and TMAO is the proatherogenic species probably promoting the associations noted between plasma levels and both prevalent and incident CVD risks.

Recent studies reveal that the potential pathogenic contribution of gut microbiota-dependent generation of TMAO may extend beyond the development of progression of atherosclerosis and its adverse complications (MI, stroke, or death). A recent observation also indicated increased TMAO levels in heart failure patients [32]. In these patients, intestinal ischaemia can be demonstrated by a decrease in intestinal mucosal pH [33] or reduced passive carrier-mediated transport of D-xylose [34]. Due to the consequences of intestinal ischaemia and congestion, the morphology, permeability, and function of the intestinal mucosa may substantially altered in congestive heart failure (CHF), especially in advanced stages with cardiac cachexia [35]. Our knowledge on the mechanistic associations between gut microbiota and CHF is improving. Although evidence is still accruing, higher concentrations of adherent bacteria have been identified in the intestinal mucosal biofilm of patients with CHF [35]. The composition of intestinal microbiota may alter rapidly during intestinal ischaemia and reperfusion or following an increase in portal vein pressure because of the activation on bacterial virulence in microbiota by gut liminal hypoxia, hypercapnia, changes in local pH, redox state, and norepinephrine [36]. Hypoperfusion and congestion in the intestine may reduce cardiac output and further disrupt the barrier function of the intestine and promote systemic inflammation through bacterial translocation, potentially leading to further CHF exacerbations (**Figure 2**). However, major changes in the gut microbial composition have not been observed in a rat model of CHF induced by coronary artery ligation [37]. In this regard, the role of gut microbiota is possibly unique to human CHF.

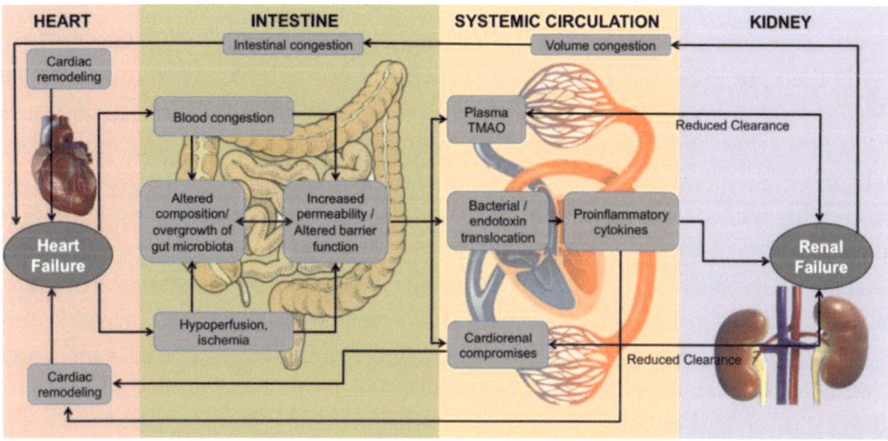

Figure 2. Links between heart failure, gut microbiota, and renal failure. The haemodynamic variations caused by heart failure affect microcirculation in intestinal villi and result in alternations of intestinal permeability and gut microbiota. The increased intestinal permeability favours microbial and endotoxin translocation, TMAO, and cardiorenal compromises can mediate the pathology that leads to further exacerbation of heart failure and renal damage. Reduced clearance of these metabolites due to impaired renal function further promotes this pathology and constitutes a vicious cycle.

The microbial analysis of atherosclerotic plaque has shown that the embedded microbiota is dominated by bacteria of the phylum *Proteobacteria* (e.g. *Escherichia coli*) [38]. *Proteobacteria* are also the most abundant microbiota in the blood of diabetic patients [39]. Hence, the establishment of microbiota might be the first step in the atherosclerotic plaque formation. Another bacterium in the genus *Collinsella* was also found to be dominant in patients with symptomatic atherosclerosis (presence of stenotic atherosclerotic plaques at the level of the carotid artery and leading to cerebrovascular episodes) The same study also indicated that there were more bacteria belonging to *Roseburia* and *Eubacterium* in the gut microbiota of healthy controls compared with patients [40]. Thus, the changes not only in microbiota composition but also in microbiome functions may be linked with the events of atherosclerosis.

3. Role of diet and host genotype in shaping intestinal microbiota profile associated with cardiovascular diseases

Dietary cholesterol has major effects on gastrointestinal microbiota, which is consequently associated with the onset of CVD. In our recent study, we tested the effect of diet and host genotype on intestinal microbiota using two Japanese quail strains that are atherosclerosis-susceptible (SUS) and atherosclerosis-resistant (RES) [41]. In that study, dietary cholesterol reduced the abundance of *Ruminococcus* and facilitated the abundance of opportunistic pathogens belonging to *Erysipelotrichaceae* in the quail ceca and may have increased the risk of assaults by these opportunistic pathogens. However, both the SUS and the RES strains housed in the same cage and fed the same high cholesterol diet hosted distinctly different ceca microbiomes.

When mice were fed a 'Western diet', which was high in fat and cholesterol, the overall diversity of their gut microbiota dropped significantly due to a bloom of a class of *Firmicutes* called *Mollicutes*, a member of which is *Eubacterium dolichum* [42]. *E. dolichum* has a number of genomic features that could promote their own fitness in competition with other microbes in the cecal nutrient metabolic milieu created by the host's consumption of the Western diet. Their abundance is associated with obesity in mice [42]. In our study, a similar situation may have occurred in RES quail in their reaction to dietary cholesterol. The ceca of RES quail were dominated by *E. dolichum* [41]. On the other hand, SUS quail fed the cholesterol diet had an abundance of *Lachnospiraceae* in the ceca [41]. At the same time, the abundance of Ruminococcaceae was not compromised [41]. *Lachnospiraceae* and *Ruminococcaceae* have been shown to be associated with the maintenance of gut health [43, 44]. These two families are specialists for degrading cellulose and hemicellulose components of plant materials, which are fermented and converted into short chain fatty acids (SCFAs) readily absorbed and used by the host [45]. SCFAs play an important role in maintaining intestinal homeostasis [43, 44]. Our study indicated that the divergent selection for susceptibility and resistance to diet-induced atherosclerosis may have adversely affected the cecal health of RES, but not SUS quail, through modification of their cecal microbiomes [41]. Whether this change in the cecal environment has effects on the metabolism and absorption of dietary cholesterol remains to be studied.

In the past decade, numerous studies have been published on the relationship between gut microbiota and cardiovascular diseases in human and in animal models. In humans, about 50% of dietary cholesterol is absorbed in the duodenum; consequently, the rest can be metabolized by *Eubacterium* bacteria to coprostanol and minor amounts of coprostanone in the large intestine [46]. Coprostanol, unlike cholesterol, is poorly absorbed by the human intestine, and hence, conversion of cholesterol to coprostanol might be a way to lower serum cholesterol in humans and rodents [47, 48]. However, feeding *Eubacterium coprostanoligenes* to laying hens did not lower plasma cholesterol levels [49]. In our study using the quail model, *E. dolichum* was found in higher abundance in the cecum of RES but not in SUS quail [41]. Although a negative correlation of *E. dolichum* abundance with plasma HDL level was significant in our study, the ability of *E. dolichum* to convert cholesterol to coprostanol has not been demonstrated. As the primary cholesterol absorption sites are in the small intestine, a comprehensive examination of the microbiota in a complete set of intestinal tract should be done to understand physiological variations at different anatomical locations of the intestinal tract, which will further elaborate the potential targets by therapeutic interventions. In the concurrent analysis on small intestinal microbiota of RES and SUS quail fed the cholesterol diet, high abundance of *Lactobacillus* species were observed in both ileum and duodenum [50] of RES but not in SUS quail. This finding is significant since *Lactobacillus* species have been proposed as an effective probiotic to lower cholesterol in humans [51].

A number of studies including our quail model highlighted the importance of host genotype in responding to diet-induced atherosclerosis. However, further research effort is need to address the underlying biochemical pathways by which host genetics interplay with diets to influence the CVD events through alteration of gut microbiota.

4. Animal models for studying gut microbiome in cardiovascular disease

Cardiovascular diseases (CVDs) involve complicated multifactorial pathologies, in which both genetic and environmental factors are involved. In order to provide us with important insights into the pathophysiology of CVD events, the development of animal models of CVD is essential as tools to evaluate novel therapeutic strategies to predict and to prevent these complications. Until now, there have been numbers of animal models used for CVD, including those implemented in both large (pig and dog) and small (mice and rat) animals, designed for enhancing scope with more precision and to better represent human pathologies. With or without genetic modifications, mouse, rat and rabbit models are more commonly used and less expensive animal models for studying CVDs compared to porcine and canine models, which better represent the human pathology, but are less popular due to the cost and difficulties in handling. For atherosclerosis, mouse models have proven to be useful to study development and progression of atherosclerotic lesions. In particular, knockout and transgenic mouse models have been well developed to study the molecular and cellular mechanisms involved in atherogenesis and to evaluate the effectiveness of new and existing drugs for the prevention and/or treatment of atherosclerosis. The most widely used knockout mouse models include low-density lipoprotein receptor-deficient mice ($LDLR^{-/-}$ mice) and apolipoprotein E-deficient mice ($ApoE^{-/-}$ mice). Mice carrying ApoE mutations such as ApoE3Leiden (E3L) and ApoE (Arg 112→Cys→142) transgenic mice are very useful mouse models to study hyperlipidaemia and atherosclerosis. The high-cholesterol diet rabbit model has been widely used for experimental atherosclerosis [52]. Several porcine models have been employed for closer representation to pathologies in humans [53–56]. However, the extensive application of porcine models is still limited. In heart failure, dog models of myocardial infarction and serial microembolization of the coronary artery were developed [57]. Like the pig models, dog models are very restricted due to their cost, ethical complications, and difficulties in handling.

Since the 'microbiome hypothesis' has been applied to CVDs and other metabolic diseases, the most common and feasible animal model is the mouse model. As we know, murine models have been extensively applied in biomedical research due to similarities in anatomy, physiology, and genetics, which have allowed numerous inferences about human pathology to be drawn from murine experimentation. In gut microbiota research, mouse models are being increasingly used to study the role and functioning of the gut microbiota and its association with diseases. However, application and direct translation of results obtained from traditional CVD mouse models to study the role of the gut microbiome and its interaction with the host have their limitations for the following reasons: [1] the variation of the gut microbiota of laboratory mice relates to genetic, physiologic, and environmental factors, and those factors also trigger the pathologies of CVD; [2] cross-talk between the gut microbiota and the host is host-specific so observations in mouse models might not be applicable to humans; [3] the inherent genetic variations in the human population cannot be captured by the inbred mouse strains that have genetic homogeneity; and finally [4] differences in multiple factors between mice and humans, such as genetic background, birth mode (caesarean or vaginal), mode of feeding (breast or bottle), diet, age, medical history, and social activities, which all contribute in shaping the gut microbiota of humans.

Existing animal models for CVDs have not yet been fully evaluated in studying the role of the gut microbiome in developing pathologies of CVD events. This should be considered in future investigations, and the most appropriate animal model to study the links between gut microbiota and CVD should be proposed and recommended. Rabbits [58], guinea pig [59], pigeon [60], and quail [61] have been used as models for studying atherosclerosis but not in association with gut microbiota. Recently, we proposed a new quail model that would be useful for studying the interaction of host genotype and diet in affecting the gut flora in association with the development of atherosclerosis [41]. We proposed that our Japanese quail model may have advantages over others because quail are naturally deficient in apolipoprotein E. When we fed a high cholesterol diet, males of the SUS quail developed lesions exhibiting structural features (e.g. focal haemorrhage, calcification, and fibrosis) that closely similar those in the human atherosclerosis [62, 63]. In addition, quail model is easier to be handled, lower costs for larger sample size, and require less laboratory space compared to other porcine or canine models. As a further incentive, our recent microbiome study has provided the baseline understanding for the association between the gut microbiome and the development of atherosclerosis in quail model.

5. The potential of modulation of gut microbiota as novel preventive and therapeutic strategies for cardiovascular disease

During these past few years, several research efforts aimed to modulate both structure and function aspects of the gut microbiome were reported [64, 65]. Faecal transplantation is one of the successful stories for restoring impaired gut microbiome into normal gut microbiome, which has shown certain success in applications of certain human diseases especially in *Clostridium difficile* infection [66]. However, several underlying questions still have not been fully resolved and more baseline information is needed. Likewise, therapeutic tools available to modulate the microbiota-driven pathogenesis of CVD remain to be validated. Besides the well-known faecal transplantation, the composition of gut microbiota can be modulated by diet, antibiotics, and prebiotic/probiotics. If we are to modulate the microbiome functions or biochemical pathways involved in microbiota-driven pathology, the crosstalk (detail mechanisms) between host and microbiota becomes a major concern, and pharmacological interventions are needed to target both host and microbiota metabolisms.

5.1. Dietary intervention

As choline, PC, and carnitine are primary sources of gut microbiota-associated TMAO production, dietary modulation is a logical intervention strategy [12]. It has been shown that vegetarians and vegans have markedly reduced production of TMA and TMAO from dietary L-carnitine and have lower plasma TMAO levels than omnivores [29]. Similarly, studies have shown that different gut microbial communities were found in vegetarians and vegans compared with omnivores [29, 67]. In animal model studies, long-term exposure to dietary L-carnitine increased TMA synthetic capacity by 10-fold with a concurrent shift in gut microbial composition [29]. Thus, chronic dietary exposure (e.g., omnivore vs. vegan/vegetarian among humans or normal chow vs. chow plus L-carnitine in mouse studies) shifts gut microbiota, with a selective advantage for certain bacterial species that prefer L-carnitine as a carbon fuel source to increase in proportion within the community and amplify the potential to produce TMA [12].

The elimination of L-carnitine from the diet is a potentially achievable goal that may reduce some TMAO production. But, choline is an essential nutrient and its complete elimination from the diet is unwise. Furthermore, bile has a very high total choline (PC) content, and the rapid turnover and sloughing of intestinal epithelial cells results in significant exposure of distal gut segments (and hence microbes) to choline, independent of dietary intake. Absorbent removal of TMA from the intestines by specific oral binding agents is a challenging but potentially feasible therapeutic approach for reducing TMA and TMAO levels. The details of application of binding reagents will be discussed in the following specific section.

5.2. Antibiotic intervention

The association between certain groups of bacteria and CVD such as atherosclerosis has previously been postulated. However, a number of randomized controlled studies have failed to demonstrate a benefit of antibiotic therapy for secondary prevention of cardiovascular events [15, 68]. On the other hand, antibiotics can influence the pathophysiological outcomes driven by changing the abundance or composition of the gut microbiota. A well-known antibiotic, vancomycin, presented a reduction of myocardial infarct size in a rat model of ischaemia-reperfusion [16]. Interestingly, there was no effect on severity of myocardial infarction by direct infusion of vancomycin into the coronary circulation. Furthermore, the oral administration of the antibiotic polymyxin B reduced monocyte production of certain proinflammatory cytokines in patients with HF and improved flow-medicated dilation [69]. Although the previous findings reflect the effect of antibiotics in the modulation of gut microbiota on the pathophysiology of various CVD events including HF, the potential adverse effects of antibiotics, such as microbial substitution and generation of antibiotic-resistant microbes, commonly occur in clinical practices. Hence, the extensive application of this strategy is arguable and challenging. Careful considerations are needed to minimize the adverse effects of antibiotic agents. Additional investigations are needed to determine the benefits of proper application of antibiotics in specific circumstances in clinical practices.

5.3. Prebiotic/probiotic intervention

Prebiotics are non-digestible food ingredients, mainly fibres that beneficially affect the host's health by selectively stimulating the growth and/or activity of some genera of gut microorganisms especially in the hindgut. Probiotics are live microorganisms that confer a health benefit to the host when administered in adequate amounts through improving the intestinal microbial balance [70]. However, the effectiveness of both prebiotics and probiotics varies on their sources, methods of preparation and administration, and the dosage. They have been extensively applied in most gastrointestinal disorders, and recently their applications in metabolic and cardiovascular diseases have been studied due to their potential role to modulate gut microbiota that consequently may diminish the pathophysiology of those diseases. In a study, done in a 'humanized' mouse model (germ-free mice colonized with human gut flora), the probiotic administration alters the production of several metabolites including TMAO through modulation of symbiotic gut microbial-host interactions [71]. Evidence has been provided that demonstrates that intervention with a probiotic product can favourably affect cardiac morphology and function in animal models [16]. A leptin suppressing probiotic bacteria, *Lactobacillus plantarum*, led to the attenuation of ischaemia-reperfusion injury in rats [16]. Additionally, in a rat myocardial infarction model, probiotic administration (*Lactobacillus rhamnosus* GR-1) reduced left ventricle (LV) hypertrophy and improved LV ejection fraction (LVEF), without colonization in the gut [37]. In HF patients, a yeast probiotic, *Saccharomyces boulardii* was shown to be beneficial by improving cardiac systolic function (LVEF) and decreasing serum creatinine and C-reactive protein (CRP) during short-term follow-up [72]. Although probiotics have generated much attention for improving CVD [37, 73], the attention on prebiotics has been limited due to its unclear definition and unfeasible applications [69]. Non-digestible beta-glucans have become one of the popular prebiotics for improving several metabolic diseases and CVD. With limited research, they have shown beneficial effects of non-digestible beta-glucans on CVD and metabolic diseases and their modulatory effect on gut microbiota (reviewed in [74]). However, long-term benefits of prebiotic and probiotic intervention strategies remain to be determined. As we described earlier in this chapter, host genotype significantly influences both the composition and probably the function of the gut microbiome, which may further interact with administered probiotics or prebiotics. Thus, the effectiveness of probiotic/prebiotic treatments may vary depending on the host genotype.

http://dx.doi.org/10.5772/64636

5.4. Binding agents of key mediators

As the metabolites (e.g. TMAO) and their precursors (e.g. TMA) play important roles in the pathogenesis of CVD, a promising intervention would be to remove such metabolites and their precursors from the gut by oral administration of specific non-absorbent binding agents. Oral charcoal absorbent (AST-120) has been clinically applied to remove uremic toxins, such as indoxyl sulphate, in patients with advanced renal failure [75]. AST-120 has been shown to prevent progression of LV hypertrophy and cardiac fibrosis in rats with chronic kidney disease (CKD) [76] and in a combination model with CKD plus HF [77] without affecting blood pressure. However, the efficacy of binding agents has not yet been demonstrated in human, and more research should explore the potential use of such strategies.

6. Conclusion

Coevolution over millions of years between human and microorganism has led to a mutualistic relationship, in which diverse ecosystems of gastrointestinal microbiota and its metabolic functions contribute to the maintenance of our metabolic homeostasis. The interaction between heart and gut, or the heart-intestine axis, has emerged as a novel concept to provide new insights into the complex mechanisms of CVD. Gut microbiota function as a filter for our largest environmental exposure, our dietary intake, and the microbial community within each of us obviously influences how we experience a diet. We need to appreciate that our gut microbial ecosystem makes up a large and plastic endocrine organ that influences numerous metabolic and physiological processes. Although recent sequencing efforts of gut microbiota provide multiple evidences of its associations with CVD events, simply cataloguing the microbes within is not sufficient and further studies should focus on discovery of the functional aspects of microbiota and its metabolites that contribute to the pathophysiology of CVD and other metabolic diseases that trigger CVD events. Not all currently available animal models are suitable for discovering the role of gut microbiota on CVD and associated diseases, thus, new *in vivo* models need to be developed and/or existing reliable models should be recommended based on their reliability and better representation of the human condition. There is increasing attention towards modulating the gut microbiota as a new target for therapeutic intervention and targeting for treatment and prevention of complex cardiometabolic diseases. However, at present time, the role of gut microbiota-targeted interventions remains ambiguous due to the absence of solid and well-documented clinical evidence. Further advances in this area have enormous potential in the development of novel therapeutic tools for microbiome modulation of CVD.

Acknowledgements

We thank the support of the British Columbia Ministry of Agriculture Specialty Birds Research Fund.

Author details

Hein Min Tun[1], Frederick C. Leung[2,3] and Kimberly M. Cheng[4*]

*Address all correspondence to: kmtc@mail.ubc.ca

1 Department of Animal Science, University of Manitoba, Winnipeg, Canada

2 School of Biological Sciences, University of Hong Kong, Hong Kong, China

3 FCL Bioscience (Hong Kong) Limited, Hong Kong Science and Technology Park, Hong Kong, China

4 Faculty of Land and Food Systems, University of British Columbia, Vancouver, Canada

References

[1] Go AS, Mozaffarian D, Roger VL, Benjamin EJ, Berry JD, Blaha MJ, et al. Heart disease and stroke statistics—2014 update: a report from the American Heart Association. Circulation. 2014;129(3):e28-e292.

[2] Nabel EG. Cardiovascular disease. The New England Journal of Medicine. 2003;349(1): 60-72.

[3] Davignon J, Ganz P. Role of endothelial dysfunction in atherosclerosis. Circulation. 2004;109(23 Suppl 1):III27-III32.

[4] Mulvihill EE, Huff MW. Citrus flavonoids and the prevention of atherosclerosis. Cardiovascular & Hematological Disorders Drug Targets. 2012;12(2):84-91.

[5] Ardissino D, Berzuini C, Merlini PA, Mannuccio Mannucci P, Surti A, Burtt N, et al. Influence of 9p21.3 genetic variants on clinical and angiographic outcomes in early-onset myocardial infarction. Journal of the American College of Cardiology. 2011;58(4): 426-434.

[6] Ripatti S, Tikkanen E, Orho-Melander M, Havulinna AS, Silander K, Sharma A, et al. A multilocus genetic risk score for coronary heart disease: case-control and prospective cohort analyses. Lancet. 2010;376(9750):1393-1400.

[7] Lozupone CA, Stombaugh JI, Gordon JI, Jansson JK, Knight R. Diversity, stability and resilience of the human gut microbiota. Nature. 2012;489(7415):220-230.

[8] Human Microbiome Project C. Structure, function and diversity of the healthy human microbiome. Nature. 2012;486(7402):207-214.

[9] Cenit MC, Matzaraki V, Tigchelaar EF, Zhernakova A. Rapidly expanding knowledge on the role of the gut microbiome in health and disease. Biochimica et Biophysica Acta. 2014;1842(10):1981-1992.

[10] Lee WJ, Hase K. Gut microbiota-generated metabolites in animal health and disease. Nature Chemical Biology. 2014;10(6):416-424.

[11] Carding S, Verbeke K, Vipond DT, Corfe BM, Owen LJ. Dysbiosis of the gut microbiota in disease. Microbial Ecology in Health and Disease. 2015;26:26191.

[12] Tang WH, Hazen SL. The contributory role of gut microbiota in cardiovascular disease. The Journal of Clinical Investigation. 2014;124(10):4204-4211.

[13] Wright SD, Burton C, Hernandez M, Hassing H, Montenegro J, Mundt S, et al. Infectious agents are not necessary for murine atherogenesis. The Journal of Experimental Medicine. 2000;191(8):1437-1442.

[14] Andraws R, Berger JS, Brown DL. Effects of antibiotic therapy on outcomes of patients with coronary artery disease: a meta-analysis of randomized controlled trials. JAMA. 2005;293(21):2641-2647.

[15] Grayston JT, Kronmal RA, Jackson LA, Parisi AF, Muhlestein JB, Cohen JD, et al. Azithromycin for the secondary prevention of coronary events. The New England Journal of Medicine. 2005;352(16):1637-1645.

[16] Lam V, Su J, Koprowski S, Hsu A, Tweddell JS, Rafiee P, et al. Intestinal microbiota determine severity of myocardial infarction in rats. FASEB Journal: official publication of the Federation of American Societies for Experimental Biology. 2012;26(4):1727-1735.

[17] McIntyre CW, Harrison LE, Eldehni MT, Jefferies HJ, Szeto CC, John SG, et al. Circulating endotoxemia: a novel factor in systemic inflammation and cardiovascular disease in chronic kidney disease. Clinical Journal of the American Society of Nephrology: CJASN. 2011;6(1):133-141.

[18] Szeto CC, Kwan BC, Chow KM, Lai KB, Chung KY, Leung CB, et al. Endotoxemia is related to systemic inflammation and atherosclerosis in peritoneal dialysis patients. Clinical Journal of the American Society of Nephrology: CJASN. 2008;3(2):431-436.

[19] Loesche WJ, Grossman NS. Periodontal disease as a specific, albeit chronic, infection: diagnosis and treatment. Clinical Microbiology Reviews. 2001;14(4):727-752, Table of contents.

[20] Blasco-Baque V, Kemoun P, Loubieres P, Roumieux M, Heymes C, Serino M, et al. Impact of periodontal disease on arterial pressure in diabetic mice. Ann Cardiol Angeiol (Paris). 2012;61(3):173-177.

[21] Bullon P, Cordero MD, Quiles JL, Morillo JM, del Carmen Ramirez-Tortosa M, Battino M. Mitochondrial dysfunction promoted by *Porphyromonas gingivalis* lipopolysacchar-

ide as a possible link between cardiovascular disease and periodontitis. Free Radical Biology & Medicine. 2011;50(10):1336-1343.

[22] Peschel T, Schonauer M, Thiele H, Anker SD, Schuler G, Niebauer J. Invasive assessment of bacterial endotoxin and inflammatory cytokines in patients with acute heart failure. European Journal of Heart Failure. 2003;5(5):609-614.

[23] Wang Z, Klipfell E, Bennett BJ, Koeth R, Levison BS, Dugar B, et al. Gut flora metabolism of phosphatidylcholine promotes cardiovascular disease. Nature. 2011;472(7341):57-63.

[24] Spencer MD, Hamp TJ, Reid RW, Fischer LM, Zeisel SH, Fodor AA. Association between composition of the human gastrointestinal microbiome and development of fatty liver with choline deficiency. Gastroenterology. 2011;140(3):976-986.

[25] Barrett EL, Kwan HS. Bacterial reduction of trimethylamine oxide. Annual Review of Microbiology. 1985;39:131-149.

[26] Zhang AQ, Mitchell SC, Smith RL. Dietary precursors of trimethylamine in man: a pilot study. Food and Chemical Toxicology: an International Journal published for the British Industrial Biological Research Association. 1999;37(5):515-520.

[27] Bain MA, Fornasini G, Evans AM. Trimethylamine: metabolic, pharmacokinetic and safety aspects. Current Drug Metabolism. 2005;6(3):227-240.

[28] Tang WH, Wang Z, Levison BS, Koeth RA, Britt EB, Fu X, et al. Intestinal microbial metabolism of phosphatidylcholine and cardiovascular risk. The New England Journal of Medicine. 2013;368(17):1575-1584.

[29] Koeth RA, Wang Z, Levison BS, Buffa JA, Org E, Sheehy BT, et al. Intestinal microbiota metabolism of l-carnitine, a nutrient in red meat, promotes atherosclerosis. Nature Medicine. 2013;19(5):576-585.

[30] Dumas ME, Barton RH, Toye A, Cloarec O, Blancher C, Rothwell A, et al. Metabolic profiling reveals a contribution of gut microbiota to fatty liver phenotype in insulin-resistant mice. Proceedings of the National Academy of Sciences of the United States of America. 2006;103(33):12511-12516.

[31] Goldsmith JR, Sartor RB. The role of diet on intestinal microbiota metabolism: downstream impacts on host immune function and health, and therapeutic implications. Journal of Gastroenterology. 2014;49(5):785-798.

[32] Simbaqueba C, Shrestha K, Patarroyo M, Troughton RW, Borowski AG, Klein AL, et al. Prognostic implications of relative hypochromia in ambulatory patients with chronic systolic heart failure. Congestive Heart Failure. 2013;19(4):180-185.

[33] Krack A, Richartz BM, Gastmann A, Greim K, Lotze U, Anker SD, et al. Studies on intragastric PCO2 at rest and during exercise as a marker of intestinal perfusion in patients with chronic heart failure. European Journal of Heart Failure. 2004;6(4):403-407.

[34] Sandek A, Bjarnason I, Volk HD, Crane R, Meddings JB, Niebauer J, et al. Studies on bacterial endotoxin and intestinal absorption function in patients with chronic heart failure. International Journal of Cardiology. 2012;157(1):80-85.

[35] Sandek A, Bauditz J, Swidsinski A, Buhner S, Weber-Eibel J, von Haehling S, et al. Altered intestinal function in patients with chronic heart failure. Journal of the American College of Cardiology. 2007;50(16):1561-1569.

[36] Alverdy J, Zaborina O, Wu L. The impact of stress and nutrition on bacterial-host interactions at the intestinal epithelial surface. Current Opinion in Clinical Nutrition and Metabolic Care. 2005;8(2):205-209.

[37] Gan XT, Ettinger G, Huang CX, Burton JP, Haist JV, Rajapurohitam V, et al. Probiotic administration attenuates myocardial hypertrophy and heart failure after myocardial infarction in the rat. Circulation Heart Failure. 2014;7(3):491-499.

[38] Koren O, Spor A, Felin J, Fak F, Stombaugh J, Tremaroli V, et al. Human oral, gut, and plaque microbiota in patients with atherosclerosis. Proceedings of the National Academy of Sciences of the United States of America. 2011;108 (Suppl. 1):4592-4598.

[39] Amar J, Serino M, Lange C, Chabo C, Iacovoni J, Mondot S, et al. Involvement of tissue bacteria in the onset of diabetes in humans: evidence for a concept. Diabetologia. 2011;54(12):3055-3061.

[40] Karlsson FH, Fak F, Nookaew I, Tremaroli V, Fagerberg B, Petranovic D, et al. Symptomatic atherosclerosis is associated with an altered gut metagenome. Nature Communications. 2012;3:1245.

[41] Liu S, Bennett DC, Tun HM, Kim JE, Cheng KM, Zhang H, et al. The effect of diet and host genotype on ceca microbiota of Japanese quail fed a cholesterol enriched diet. Frontiers in Microbiology. 2015;6:1092.

[42] Turnbaugh PJ, Backhed F, Fulton L, Gordon JI. Diet-induced obesity is linked to marked but reversible alterations in the mouse distal gut microbiome. Cell Host & Microbe. 2008;3(4):213-223.

[43] Pryde SE, Duncan SH, Hold GL, Stewart CS, Flint HJ. The microbiology of butyrate formation in the human colon. FEMS Microbiology Letters. 2002;217(2):133-139.

[44] Greer RL, Morgun A, Shulzhenko N. Bridging immunity and lipid metabolism by gut microbiota. The Journal of Allergy and Clinical Immunology. 2013;132(2):253-262; quiz 63.

[45] Biddle A, Stewart L, Blanchard J, Leschine S. Untangling the genetic basis of fibrolytic specialization by Lachnospiraceae and Ruminococcaceae in diverse gut communities. Diversity. 2013;5(3):627-640.

[46] Macdonald IA, Bokkenheuser VD, Winter J, McLernon AM, Mosbach EH. Degradation of steroids in the human gut. Journal of Lipid Research. 1983;24(6):675-700.

[47] Stepankova R, Tonar Z, Bartova J, Nedorost L, Rossman P, Poledne R, et al. Absence of microbiota (germ-free conditions) accelerates the atherosclerosis in ApoE-deficient mice fed standard low cholesterol diet. Journal of Atherosclerosis and Thrombosis. 2010;17(8):796-804.

[48] Sekimoto H, Goto Y, Goto Y, Naito C, Yasugi T, Okido M, et al. Changes of serum total cholesterol and triglyceride levels in normal subjects in Japan in the past twenty years. Research committee on familial hyperlipidemia in Japan. Japanese Circulation Journal. 1983;47(12):1351-1358.

[49] Li L, Baumann CA, Meling DD, Sell JL, Beitz DC. Effect of orally administered *Eubacterium coprostanoligenes* ATCC 51222 on plasma cholesterol concentration in laying hens. Poultry Science. 1996;75(6):743-745.

[50] Liu S, Tun HM, Bennett DC, Leung FC, Zhang H, Cheng KM. Interaction of genotype and diet on atherosclerosis development and bacterial dysbiosis in the small intestine of Japanese quail fed a cholesterol enriched diet. Frontiers in Microbiology. 2016 (Manuscript in prep).

[51] Jones ML, Martoni CJ, Prakash S. Cholesterol lowering and inhibition of sterol absorption by *Lactobacillus reuteri* NCIMB 30242: a randomized controlled trial. European Journal of Clinical Nutrition. 2012;66(11):1234-1241.

[52] Hofker MH, van Vlijmen BJ, Havekes LM. Transgenic mouse models to study the role of APOE in hyperlipidemia and atherosclerosis. Atherosclerosis. 1998;137(1):1-11.

[53] Molacek J, Treska V, Kobr J, Certik B, Skalicky T, Kuntscher V, et al. Optimization of the model of abdominal aortic aneurysm--experiment in an animal model. Journal of Vascular Research. 2009;46(1):1-5.

[54] Gerrity RG, Natarajan R, Nadler JL, Kimsey T. Diabetes-induced accelerated atherosclerosis in swine. Diabetes. 2001;50(7):1654-1665.

[55] Granada JF, Kaluza GL, Wilensky RL, Biedermann BC, Schwartz RS, Falk E. Porcine models of coronary atherosclerosis and vulnerable plaque for imaging and interventional research. EuroIntervention: Journal of EuroPCR in Collaboration with the Working Group on Interventional Cardiology of the European Society of Cardiology. 2009;5(1):140-148.

[56] Hamada N, Miyata M, Eto H, Shirasawa T, Akasaki Y, Nagaki A, et al. Tacrolimus-eluting stent inhibits neointimal hyperplasia via calcineurin/NFAT signaling in porcine coronary artery model. Atherosclerosis. 2010;208(1):97-103.

[57] Lavine SJ. Effect of changes in contractility on the index of myocardial performance in the dysfunctional left ventricle. Cardiovascular Ultrasound. 2006;4:45.

[58] Shiomi M, Yamada S, Matsukawa A, Itabe H, Ito T. Invasion of atheromatous plaques into tunica media causes coronary outward remodeling in WHHLMI rabbits. Atherosclerosis. 2008;198(2):287-293.

[59] Fernandez ML, Volek JS. Guinea pigs: a suitable animal model to study lipoprotein metabolism, atherosclerosis and inflammation. Nutrition & Metabolism. 2006;3:17.

[60] Anderson JL, Ashwell CM, Smith SC, Shine R, Smith EC, Taylor RL, Jr. Atherosclerosis-susceptible and atherosclerosis-resistant pigeon aortic cells express different genes in vivo. Poultry Science. 2013;92(10):2668-2680.

[61] Chapman KP, Stafford WW, Day CE. Produced by selective breeding of Japanese quail animal model for experimental atherosclerosis. Advances in Experimental Medicine and Biology. 1976;67(00):347-356.

[62] Shih JC, Pullman EP, Kao KJ. Genetic selection, general characterization, and histology of atherosclerosis-susceptible and -resistant Japanese quail. Atherosclerosis. 1983;49(1): 41-53.

[63] Haust MD. The natural history of human atherosclerotic lesions. In: Moore S, editor. Vascular Injury and Atherosclerosis. New York: Marcell Dekker; 1981. p. 1-23.

[64] Walsh CJ, Guinane CM, O'Toole PW, Cotter PD. Beneficial modulation of the gut microbiota. FEBS Letters. 2014;588(22):4120-4130.

[65] Rajpal DK, Brown JR. Modulating the human gut microbiome as an emerging therapeutic paradigm. Science Progress. 2013;96(Pt 3):224-236.

[66] Cammarota G, Ianiro G, Gasbarrini A. Fecal microbiota transplantation for the treatment of *Clostridium difficile* infection: a systematic review. Journal of Clinical Gastroenterology. 2014;48(8):693-702.

[67] David LA, Maurice CF, Carmody RN, Gootenberg DB, Button JE, Wolfe BE, et al. Diet rapidly and reproducibly alters the human gut microbiome. Nature. 2014;505(7484): 559-563.

[68] Cannon CP, Braunwald E, McCabe CH, Grayston JT, Muhlestein B, Giugliano RP, et al. Antibiotic treatment of *Chlamydia pneumoniae* after acute coronary syndrome. The New England Journal of Medicine. 2005;352(16):1646-1654.

[69] Conraads VM, Jorens PG, De Clerck LS, Van Saene HK, Ieven MM, Bosmans JM, et al. Selective intestinal decontamination in advanced chronic heart failure: a pilot trial. European Journal of Heart Failure. 2004;6(4):483-491.

[70] de Vrese M, Schrezenmeir J. Probiotics, prebiotics, and synbiotics. Advances in Biochemical Engineering/Biotechnology. 2008;111:1-66.

[71] Martin FP, Wang Y, Sprenger N, Yap IK, Lundstedt T, Lek P, et al. Probiotic modulation of symbiotic gut microbial-host metabolic interactions in a humanized microbiome mouse model. Molecular Systems Biology. 2008;4:157.

[72] Costanza AC, Moscavitch SD, Faria Neto HC, Mesquita ET. Probiotic therapy with *Saccharomyces boulardii* for heart failure patients: a randomized, double-blind, placebo-controlled pilot trial. International Journal of Cardiology. 2015;179:348-350.

[73] Kumar M, Nagpal R, Kumar R, Hemalatha R, Verma V, Kumar A, et al. Cholesterol-lowering probiotics as potential biotherapeutics for metabolic diseases. Experimental Diabetes Research. 2012;2012:902917.

[74] Kumar H, Salminen S, Verhagen H, Rowland I, Heimbach J, Banares S, et al. Novel probiotics and prebiotics: road to the market. Current Opinion in Biotechnology. 2015;32:99-103.

[75] Mosinska P, Storr M, Fichna J. The role of AST-120 and protein-bound uremic toxins in irritable bowel syndrome: a therapeutic perspective. Therapeutic Advances in Gastroenterology. 2015;8(5):278-284.

[76] Lekawanvijit S, Kompa AR, Manabe M, Wang BH, Langham RG, Nishijima F, et al. Chronic kidney disease-induced cardiac fibrosis is ameliorated by reducing circulating levels of a non-dialysable uremic toxin, indoxyl sulfate. PLoS One. 2012;7(7):e41281.

[77] Fujii H, Nishijima F, Goto S, Sugano M, Yamato H, Kitazawa R, et al. Oral charcoal adsorbent (AST-120) prevents progression of cardiac damage in chronic kidney disease through suppression of oxidative stress. Nephrology, Dialysis, Transplantation: official publication of the European Dialysis and Transplant Association—European Renal Association. 2009;24(7):2089-2095.

Section 5

Gut Flora and Therapeutic Possibilities

Chapter 5

Gut Flora: In the Treatment of Disease

Sonia B. Bhardwaj

Additional information is available at the end of the chapter

http://dx.doi.org/10.5772/65073

Abstract

Gut flora is the largest reservoir of human flora. It is an essential factor in certain pathological disorders, including multisystem organ failure, colon cancer and inflammatory bowel diseases and extraintestinal disorders, such as allergy, asthma and even obesity. Prebiotics and probiotics are known to have a role in prevention or treatment of some diseases. Nevertheless, bacteria have been found to be useful for treating disease and thus promoting human health in a safe and natural way.

Keywords: gut flora, cancer, allergy, inflammatory bowel disease, obesity

1. Introduction

The endogenous gastrointestinal microbial flora plays a fundamentally important role in normal health and disease [1]. According to recent advances in microbiome research, the infectious, inflammatory and functional bowel diseases are closely associated with the pathologic changes in gut microbiota. Recent discovery of the fact that disbalance of gut microbiome has a profound impact on the function of the liver through microbiota liver axis [2]. There has been a re-emergence of interest in the relationship between gastrointestinal flora and gut function with the recognition that prebiotics, probiotics and other means of modifying gut flora may function as therapeutic modalities.

2. The normal flora

The human intestine is colonized by millions of bacteria, primarily anaerobic bacteria, comprising approximately 1000 species. The bacterial distribution varies greatly at different

INTECH
open science | open minds

© 2016 The Author(s). Licensee InTech. This chapter is distributed under the terms of the Creative Commons Attribution License (http://creativecommons.org/licenses/by/3.0), which permits unrestricted use, distribution, and reproduction in any medium, provided the original work is properly cited. (cc) BY

levels of the gastrointestinal tract (GIT) [2] ranging from <10^3 colony-forming units/ml (CFU/ml) in the stomach to 10^{11}–10^{12} CFU/ml within the colon, where anaerobes outnumber aerobes by a ratio of 1000:1.

2.1. Types of flora

2.1.1. Commensal flora

The intestinal flora includes Bifidobacteria, Lactobacillus, Propionobacteria, Peptostreptococci and Enterococci. The commensal flora produces antibiotic-like substances that are anti-fungal, anti-viral and reduce pH near the wall of the gut forming a protective barrier, which is uninhabitable for the pathogenic bacteria to colonize [3].

2.1.2. Opportunistic flora

This includes intestinal flora like Bacteroides, Peptococci, Staphylococci, Streptococci, Bacilli, Clostridia, Yeasts, Enterobacteria, Fusobacteria, Eubacteria, Catenobacteria and others. In a healthy person, their numbers are limited and controlled by commensal flora.

2.1.3. Transitional Flora

The flora which enters the body through food and drink constitutes the transitional flora. In a healthy gut microbiome, it does not cause disease however any harm to the commensal flora will enable them to cause the disease.

3. Role of gut flora in the treatment of disease

3.1. Cancer

Indiscriminate use of antibiotics not only makes the problem of antibiotic resistant bacterial strains even worse, but also kills many commensal bacteria that promote homeostasis and protect against carcinogenesis. It has been seen that changes in the bacterial community occur in the gut microbiome of colon cancer patients, with tumors harboring increased bacterial diversity and an abundance of pathogenic bacteria compared to surrounding healthy tissue [4]. Lactobacillus and Bifidobacteria are known to prevent tumor formation by suppressing the growth factors like MyD88 (an adaptor molecule necessary for most toll-like receptors (TLR) signaling) was found to be essential in the development of the carcinomas [5, 6].

A number of *in vitro* and animal studies provide evidence that consuming probiotics suppresses colon rectal cancer. These studies have also proposed multiple pathways by which probiotics could inhibit colon cancer by influencing innate immune pathways and apoptosis, reducing oxidative stress and modulating intestinal bacteria and their metabolism [7]. *Lactobacillus johnsonii* reduced the concentration of *Enterobacters* and modulated immune response in colon rectal cancer patients, whereas *Bifidobacterium longum* did not have any effect.

In another study, *L. casei* suppressed colorectal tumor growth in patients, after 2–4 years of treatment. However, these clinical trials are limited by the small number of subjects and their short duration [8]. Mice experimentally colonized with *Helicobacter hepaticus* and enterotoxigenic *Bacteroides fragilis* exhibit colonic Th17 inflammatory infiltrates that appear to have a beneficial role in human ovarian cancer [9], murine melanoma, pancreatic and colon cancer [10–12]. It has also been found that *Helicobacter pylori* can alter stomach pH and acid reflux, which could protect against Barrett's esophagus and esophageal cancer [13].

4. Probiotics and prebiotics in cancer prevention

Fecal microbiota transplantations (FMT) are effective in maintaining a healthy gut microbiome particularly in patients with severe *Clostridium difficile* infections. A recent study transplanted a culture of six phylogenetically diverse gut microbes into mice. With *C. difficile* infections, this restored a normal microbial community, displaced the *Clostridium difficile* and resolved the disease [14].

Probiotics are live microorganisms present in foods as dietary supplement that confer a health benefit. Lactobacilli in yoghurt improved digestion of dairy products in individuals who are lactose intolerant [15]. Probiotics can be improved upon by supplementing food with bacteria engineered to have more beneficial effect. Oral administration of a strain of *Lactobacillus acidophilus* (having phosphoglycerol transferase gene deleted) to APC floxed mice resulted in the reduction in polyps [16]. A protein elafin produced by engineered strains of *Lactobacillus casie* and *Lactococcus lactis* diminished inflammation in a mouse model of colitis [17]. Another example is a strain of *Lactobacillus gasseri*, which was engineered to overexpress the antioxidant superoxide dismutase and decreased colitis in interleukin (IL)-10 knockout mice [18]. The introduction of genetically engineered organisms to produce and deliver cytokines or other biologically relevant molecules to the mucosa offers further potential to the probiotics.

Prebiotics are the non-digestible food ingredient that beneficially affects the host by stimulating the growth or activity of a genus of bacteria. A number of prebiotics have been implicated in cancer prevention [19]. Prebiotics include dietary fiber sources such as inulin that promote the growth of bifidobacteria. Dietary polyphenols include flavonoids, phenolic acids, lignins present in tea, wine, fruits, nuts and vegetables. Ellagic acid is polyphenol present in certain berries and nuts that is an antioxidant with cancer preventive properties [20]. Epidemiological studies have reported correlations between equol or equol-producing bacteria and diminished breast cancer risk in women and diminished prostate cancer in men in Asian populations [21].

However, further studies are needed to determine whether probiotics can be used as protective agents for the prevention of human colon cancer. It is possible that a microbiota favoring commensal bacteria could alter the immune response to tumors at extraintestinal as well as intestinal sites.

5. Treatment of inflammatory bowel disease and colitis

Bacterial species isolated from inflammatory bowel disease (IBD) patients have shown to be capable of inducing intestinal inflammation (e.g., enterotoxigenic *B. fragilis, Bacteroides vulgates*). Intestinal inflammation was seen in germ-free SCID mice colonized with individual or combinations of strains of *Enterococcus faecalis, Fusobacterium mortiferum, Bacteroides distasonis* and segmented filamentous bacteria (SFB) [22]. SFB also play a role in the development of experimental autoimmune encephalomyelitis (EAE) [23] and Rheumatoid arthritis(RA) [24]. Because of the potentially harmful role of these bacteria, antibiotics are frequently prescribed to treat IBD [25].

A probiotic nonpathogenic strain of *E.coli* has been shown to be effective in patients diagnosed with ulcerative colitis [26]. More recently, a probiotic product called VSL#3 which is a combination of eight probiotics: *Bifidobacterium breve, B. longum, Bifidobacterium infantis, L. acidophilus, Lactobacillus plantarum, Lactobacillus paracasei, Lactobacillus bulgaricus* and *Streptococcus thermophilus* have demonstrated efficacy for inducing remission in ulcerative colitis [27].

6. Fecal microbiota transplantation and IBD

The results of fecal microbiota transplantation (FMT) show very promising but discrepant results. A meta-analysis recently conducted by Colman *et al.* showed that 45% of patients achieved clinical remission and reduced some anti-inflammatory drugs after FMT [28–30]. A recently conducted randomized trial in patients with ulcerative colitis showed that the clinical remission was not statistically significant with FMT due to small study numbers but in all the responders a shift in the microbiota composition was observed supporting the role of microbiota manipulation in the treatment of IBD [31, 32].

7. Helminth: induced suppression of IBD

Novel treatment strategies for IBD and celiac disease are being developed using parasitic nematodes particularly *Trichuris* spp. and *Necator americanus* [33, 34].

Studies of the impact of parasite colonization on the human gut microbiota have shed light on the potential role of the gut microbiota in whipworm-mediated suppression of inflammation. The therapeutic ability of *T. trichura* whipworms to improve clinical symptoms of inflammation associated with significant changes in the composition and relative abundance of different gut bacterial species has been shown [35]. A significant decrease in the bacterial phylum cyanobacteria accompanied by an expansion of Bacteroidetes and Tenericutes was seen in Trichuris-infected ICD macques. In another study, the administration of a single dose of *T. suis* ova was able to alter the composition of the gut microbiota of infected pigs with IBD, including a reduction in the abundance of Fibrobacter and Ruminococcus expansion of Campylobacter [36].

Another study involving experimental infection with *Heligmosomoides polygyrus bakeri* in a mouse model of IBD revealed a significant expansion of the bacterial family Lactobacillaceae in the ileum of infected mice, which correlated with disease outcome [37].

8. Therapeutic potential of Hookworms

While heavy burdens of hookworm parasites are associated with pathological effects, experimental infections with small numbers of *N. americanus* are safe and well tolerated. When administered in a mouse model of IBD, hookworm excretory/secretory products protect against inflammation and weight loss [38]. A pilot study done to explore the impact of experimental infections with *N. americanus* on the human gut microbiota has shown increased bacterial richness at 8 weeks post infection in the volunteer subjects [39]. A higher species richness of the gut microbiota has been associated with healthier homeostasis.

9. Role of microbiota in allergic diseases

Allergic disease development has been associated with alterations in the intestinal microbiota. Infants with food allergies were found to exhibit lower lactobacilli and bifidobacteria species while coliforms and *Staphylococcus aureus* were higher [40]. Bifidobacteria was decreased while increase in clostridia was found in infants with atopic dermatitis [41]. Administration of *L. casei* GG to the mothers before and after delivery prevents atopic eczema, which develop later in children at risk [42]. A number of studies have been performed using probiotics to treat the severity of various allergic diseases, including atopic eczema, atopic dermatitis and food allergy in these children [43, 44]. Oral administration of optimal combinations of probiotic Lactobacilli and Bifidobacteria in murine models is able to reduce allergic diseases. This could be due to lower Th2 cytokine secretion on innate exposure [45, 46].

Environmental exposures in early infancy are thus a deciding factor of the composition of gut microbiota which decides the development of immune function in an individual. These differences in immune function link to the development of allergy and asthma [47].

A possible interpretation is that the bacteria ingested or inhaled served as a kind of tolerance inducing adjuvant for allergens ingested or inhaled as reported recently that commensal bacteria protect against food allergen sensitization [48]. The bacteria associated with protection were largely members of the Bacteriodetes and Firmicutes phyla (e.g., Rickenellaceae, Porphyromonadaceae, Lachnospiraceae, Prevotellaceae, etc.).

Several associations exist between commensal microbiota and the development of allergic diseases. In prospective studies, early fecal samples of infants who go on to develop allergies, compared to those who remain healthy, grew less Enterococci, Bifidobacteria, Bacteroides, Clostridia and Staphylococci [49]. Japanese infants developing early allergy have different *bifidobacteria* spp compared to nonallergic infants [50]. In an experimental animal model of food allergy, the gut microbiota and its stimulatory action on innate immune system by toll-like receptors (TLR), particularly TLR4, have been found. Mice susceptible to food allergies have a mutation in TLR4 blocking its signaling [51].

10. Mode of action of probiotics to treat/prevent allergy

Probiotics have been suggested to act by reducing the permeability of intestine [52]. Probiotics induce low grade inflammation characterized by increases in CRP, total IgA, total IgE and IL-10 levels. They can interact with the host immune system and modify the natural course of allergic disease [53]. Recent data indicate that probiotics could modulate the production of cytokines by monocytes and lymphocytes [54]. The dendritic cells may be stimulated by probiotic bacteria in the intestinal lumen and express TLR-2 and inflammatory cytokines [55]. Therefore, the stimulation of innate immunity may be the cause of the observed inflammatory signs and beneficial clinical effects.

11. Role of microflora in obesity

The microbes occupying the human gut are in direct relation to obesity. The obese have more Firmicutes and fewer Bacteroidetes. The more Bacteroidetes, the more weight loss by an obese person [56]. An opportunistic pathogen isolated from the gut of obese human causing obesity in germ-free mice has been identified [57].

Housing mice with obese microbiota with those of lean microbiota suppresses the obesity factor in the former mice [58]. These data indicate clearly that microbiota can influence metabolic parameters or even obesity [59, 60].

12. Regulation of obesity by gut flora

12.1. Extraction of addition calories from ingested food

The intestinal flora of obese individuals has been suggested to undergo changes that would increase the extraction of calories from nutrients. An animal study, using germ-free mice observed that these mice despite ingesting greater amounts of food than conventionally raised mice, presented a lower amount of body fat [61]. Another study has shown that obese mice had a reduced number of Bacteroides and a proportional increase in Firmicutes when compared to lean mice [62]. They also proposed that flora of obese mice favored a greater capacity of extracting calories from food, as the feces of these mice were observed to have less calories and a greater amount of fermentation end products.

http://dx.doi.org/10.5772/65073

12.2. Induction of subclinical inflammation

A correlation between obesity and intestinal flora has been proposed in type 2 diabetes. The inflammation that leads to diabetes in obesity has been proposed to be triggered by LPS of Gram-negative bacteria, which compose the intestinal flora [63]. Also it has been seen that in humans, individuals with type 2 diabetes presented lower levels of serum lipopolysaccharide than patients with type 2 diabetes by age [64]. Also in animal studies, it has been seen that mice treated with a high fat diet were observed to present a reduction in intestinal permeability and in serum LPS levels, in addition to a decrease in inflammation of adipose tissue and macrophage infiltration, after the modification of gut flora by antibiotics [65].

13. Conclusion

The endogenous gastrointestinal flora plays a fundamentally important role in health and disease. The characterization of this diverse ecosystem fuelled by the recognition of the potential value of probiotics and other means of modifying gut flora can be used as future therapeutic modalities. It may hence be possible to establish profiles of the microbiota in humans based on the bacterial species composition of the enterotypes [66].

Author details

Sonia B. Bhardwaj

Address all correspondence to: sbbhardwaj2002@yahoo.com

Panjab University, Chandigarh, India

References

[1] Hooper LV, Gordon JI. Commensal host-bacterial relationships in the gut. Science 2001; 292:1115–1118.

[2] Mondot S, de Wouters T, Dore J, Lepage P. The human gut microbiome and its dysfunctions. Dig Dis Sci 2013; 31:278–285.

[3] Szabo G. Gut—liver axis in alcoholic liver disease. Gastroenterology 2015; 148:30–36.

[4] Simon GL, Gorbach SL. Intestinal flora in health and disease. Gastroenterology 1984; 86:174–193.

[5] Borrielio SP. Microbial flora of the gastrointestinal tract. In Microbial Metabolism in the Digestive Tract. Hill MJ (ed), CRC Press Inc, Boca Raton, FL, 1986; 2–19.

[6] O' Keefe SJ, Ou J, Aufreiter S, O' Connor D, Sharma S, Sepulveda J, Fukuwatari T, Shibata K, Mawhinney T. Products of the colonic microbiota mediate the effects of diet on colon cancer risk. J Nutr 2009; 139:2044–2048.

[7] Challa A, Rao DR, Chawan CB, Shackelford L. Bifidobacterium longum and lactulose suppress azoxymethane- induced colonic aberrant crypt foci in rats. Carcinogenesis 1997; 18:517–521.

[8] Rowland IR, Rumney CJ, Coutts JT, Lievense LC. Effect of Bifidobacterium longum and Inulin on gut bacterial metabolism and carcinogen induced aberrant crypt foci in rats. Carcinogenesis 1998; 19:281–285.

[9] Ishikawa H, Akedo I, Otani T, Suzuki T, Nakamura T, Takeyama I, Ishiguro S, Miyaoka E, Sobus T, Kakizoe T. Randomised trial of dietary fiber and Lactobacillus casei administration for prevention of colorectal tumors. Int J Cancer 2005; 116:762–767.

[10] Kearney J, Giovannuci E, Rimm EB, Ascherio A, Stampfer MJ, Colditz GA, Wing A, Kampman E, Willet WC. Calcium, vitamin D and dairy foods and the occurrence of colon cancer in men. Am J Epidemiol 1996; 143:907–917.

[11] Kryczek I, Banerjee M, Cheng P, Vatan L, Szelgia W, Wei S, Huang E, Finlayson E, Simeone D, Welling TH, Chang A, Coukos G, Liu R, Zou W. Phenotype, distribution, generation, and functional and clinical relevance of Th17 cells in the human tumor environments. Blood 2009; 114: 1141–1149.

[12] Muranski P, Boni A, Antony PA, Cassard L, Irvine KR, Kaiser A, Paulos CM, Palmer DC, Touloukian CS, Kerstann KW, Freigenbaum L, Chan CC, Restifo NP. Tumor specific Th17-polarized cells eradicate large established melanoma. Blood 2008; 112:362–373.

[13] Gnerlich JL, Mitchem JB, Weir JS, Sankpal NV, Kashiwagi H, Belt BA, Porembka MR, Herndon JM, Eberlein TJ, Goedgebure P, Linehan DC. Induction of Th17 cells in the tumor microenvironment improves survival in a murine model of pancreatic cancer. J Immunol 2010; 185:4063–4071.

[14] Kryzek I, Wei S, Szelgia W, Vatan L, Zou W. Endogenous IL-17 contributes to reduced tumor growth and metastasis. Blood 2009; 114:357–359.

[15] Blaser M. Antibiotic overuse: stop killing of beneficial bacteria. Nature 2011; 476: 393–394.

[16] Lawley TD, Clare S, Walker AW, Stares MD, Connor TR. Targeted restoration of the intestinal microbiota with a simple, defined bacteriotherapy resolves relapsing C. difficile disease in mice. PLoS Pathog 2012; 8: e1002995.

[17] Guarner F, Malagelada JR. Gut flora in health and disease. Lancet 2003;361:512–519.

[18] Khazaie K, Zadeh M, Khan MW, Bere P, Gounari F, Dennis K, Blatner NR, Jennifer L, Owen LJR, Klaenhamme TR, Mohamadzadeh M. Abating colon cancer polyposis by

Lactobacillus acidophilus deficient in lipoteichoic acid. Proc Natl Acad Sci 2012; 109:10462–10467.

[19] Motta JP, Bermudez-Humaran LG, Deraison C, Martin L, Rolland C, Rousset P, Boue J, Dietrich G, Chapman K, Kharrat P, Vinel JP, Alric L, Mass E, Sallenave JM, Langella P, Vergnolle N. Food grade bacteria expressing elafin protect against inflammation and restore colon homeostasis. Sci Transl Med 2012;4:158 ra 144.

[20] Carroll I M, Andrus JM, Bruno-Bárcena JM Klaaenhammer TR, Hassan HM, Threadgill DS. Anti-inflammatory properties of Lactobacillus gassei expressing manganese superoxide dismutase using the interleukin 10-deficient mice model of colitis. Am J Physiol Gastrointest Liver Physiol 2007; 293:G729–G738.

[21] Larrosa M, González-Sarrías A, García-Conesa MT, Tomás-Barberán FA, Espín JC. Urolithins, ellagic acid derived metabolites produced by human colonic microflora, exhibit estrogenic and anti estrogenic activities. J Agric Food Chem 2006; 54:1611–1620.

[22] González-Sarrías A, Larrosa M, Tomás-Barberán FA, Dolara P, Espín JC. NF-Kappa B dependant anti-inflammatory activity of urolithins, gut microbiota ellagic acid-derived metabolites in human colonic fibroblasts. Br J Nutr 2010;104:503–512.

[23] Lampe JW. Emerging research on equol and cancer. J Nutr 2010; 140:1369S–1372S.

[24] Feng T, Wang L, Schoeb TR, Elson CO, Cong Y. Microbiota innate stimulation is a prerequisite for T cell spontaneous proliferation and induction of experimental colitis. J Exp Med 2010; 207:1321–1332.

[25] Lee YK, Menzes JS, Umesaki Y, Mazmanian SK. Proinflammatory T cell responses to gut microbiota promote experimental autoimmune encephalomyelitis. Proc Natl Acad Sci USA 2011; 108(Supp.1):4615–4622.

[26] Wu HJ, Ivanov Li, Darce J, Hattori K, Shima T, Umesaki Y, Littman DR, Benoist C, Mathis D. Gut—residing segmented filamentous bacteria drive autoimmune arthritis via T helper 17 cells. Immunity 2010; 32:815–827.

[27] Suenaert P, Bulteel V, Lemmens L, Noman M, Geypens B, Van Assche G, Geboes K, Ceuppens JL, Rutgeerts P. Anti-tumor necrosis factor treatment restores the gut barrier in Crohn's disease. Am J Gastroenterol 2002; 97:2000–2004.

[28] Rembacken BJ, Snelling AM, Hawkey PM, Chalmers DM, Axon AT. Non-pathogenic Escherichia coli versus mesalazine for the treatment of ulcerative colitis, a randomized trial. Lancet 1999;354(9179):635–639.

[29] Gionchetti P, Rizzello F, Venturi A, Brigidi P, Matteuzzi D, Bazzocchi G, Poggioli G, Miglioli M, Campieri M. Oral bacteriotherapy as maintenance treatment in patients with chronic pouchitis: a double blind placebo controlled trial. Gastroenterology 2000; 119:305–309.

[30] Colman RJ, Rubin DT. Fecal microbiota transplantation as therapy for IBD: a systematic review and meta-analysis. J Crohn's Colitis 2014; 8:1569–1581.

[31] Kruis W, Fric P, Stolte M. Maintenance of remission in ulcerative colitis is equally effective with Escherichia coli Nissle 1917 and with standard mesalamine. Gastroenterology 2001; 120(5):A127–A127 (Abstract).

[32] Rossen NG, Fuentes S, van der Spek MJ, Tijssen JG. Rossen N, Fuentes S. Findings from randomized controlled trial of fecal transplantation for patients with ulcerative colitis. Gastroenterology 2015; 149:110–118.

[33] Weinstock JV, Elliot DE. Translatability of helminth therapy in IBD. Int J Parasitol 2013; 43:245–251.

[34] Croese J, Gaze ST, Loukas A. Changed gluten immunity in celiac disease by Necator americanus provides new insights into autoimmunity. Int J Parasitol 2013; 43:275–282.

[35] Broadhurst J, Adeshir A, Kanwar B, Mirpuri J, Gundra UM, Leung JM, Wiens KE, Vujkovic-Cvijin I,. Kim CC, Yarovinsky F, Lerche NW. McCune JM, P'ng Loke. Therapeutic helminth infection of macques with idiopathic chronic diarrhea alters the inflammatory signature and mucosal microbiota of the colon. PLoS Pathog 2012; 8:e1003000.

[36] Wu S, Lir W, Beshah E, Dawson HD, Urban JF Jr. Worm burden dependent disruption of the porcine colon microbiota by Trichuris suis infection. PLoS One 2012; 7:e35470.

[37] Reynolds, L. A., K. A. Smith, K. J. Filbey, Y. Harcus, J. P. Hewitson, S. A. Redpath, Y. Valdez, M. J. Yebra, B. B. Finlay, and R. M. Maizels. Commensal-pathogsen interactions in the intestinal tract: lactobacilli promote infection with, and are promoted by, helminth parasites. Gut Microbes, 2014, 5: 522–532.

[38] Ferreira I et al. Hookworm excretory/secretory products induce interleukin 4 (IL-4), IL-10, CD4+ T cell responses and suppress pathology in a mouse model of colitis. Infect Immun 2013; 81:2104–2111.

[39] Cantessi I, Giacomin P, Croese J, Zakrzewski M, Sotillo J, McCann L, Nolan MJ, Mitreva M, Krause L, Loukas A. Impact of experimental hookworm infection on the human gut microbiota. J infect Dis 2014; 10:1431–1434.

[40] Beasley B, Crane I, Lai CK, Pearce N. Prevalence and etiology of asthma. J Allergy Clin Immunol 2000; 105:S466–S472.

[41] Bjorksten B, Selep Mikelsaar M. Allergy development and the intestinal flora during the first year of life. J Allergy Clin Immunol 2001; 108:516–520.

[42] Kalliomaki M, Salminen S, Poussa T, Arvillommi H, Isolauri E. Probiotics and prevention of atopic disease: 4 year follow up of a randomized placebo-controlled trial. Lancet 2003; 361:1869–1871.

[43] Rosenfeldt V, Benfeldt E, Nielsen SD, Michaelsen KF, Jeppesen DL, Valerius NH, Paerregaard A. Effect of probiotic Lactobacillus strains in children with atopic dermatitis. J Allergy Clin Immunol 2003; 111:389–395.

[44] Viljanen M, Savilahti E, Haahtela T, Juntunen-Backman K, Korpela R, Possa T, Tuure T, Kuitunen M. Probiotics in the treatment atopic eczema/dermatitis syndrome in infants: a double-blind placebo-controlled trial. Allergy 2005; 60:494–500.

[45] Karimi K, Inman MD, Bienstock J, Forsythe P. Lactobacillus reuteri-induced regulatory T cells protect against an allergic airway response in mice. Am J Respir Crit Care Med 2009; 179:186–193.

[46] Lyons A, O'Mahony D, O'Brien F, Macsharry J, Sheil B, Ceddia M, Russell WM, Forsythe P, Bienenstock J, Kiely B, Shanahan F, O'Mahony L. Bacterial strain-specific induction of Foxp3+ T regulatory cells is protective in murine allergy models. Clin Exp Allergy models 2010; 40:811–819.

[47] Gollwitzer ES, Saglani S, Trompette A, Yadava K, Sherburn R, McCoy KD, Nicod LP, Lloyd CM, Marsland B. Lung microbiota promotes tolerance to allergens in neonates via PD L1. Nat Med 2014; 20:642–647.

[48] Stefka AT, Feehley T, Tripathi P, Qiu J, McCoy K, Mazmanian SK, Tjota MY, Seo GY, Cao S, Theriault BR, Antonopoulos DA, Zhou L, Chang EB, Fu YX, Nagler CR. Commensal bacteria protect against food allergen sensitization. Proc Natl Acad Sci USA 2014; 111:13145–13150.

[49] Bjorksten B, Stepp E, Julge K, Voor T, Mikelsaar M. Allergy development and the intestinal microflora during the first year of life. J Allergy Clin Immunol 2001; 108:516–520.

[50] Suzuki S, Shimojo N, Tajiri Y, Kumemura M, Kohno Y. Differences in composition of intestinal Bifidobacterium species and the development of allergic diseases in infants in rural Japan. Clin Exp Allergy 2007; 37:507–511.

[51] Poltorak A, He X, Smirnova I, Liv MY, Van Huffel C, Du X, Birdwell D, Alejos E, Silva M, Galanos C, Freudenberg M, Ricciardi-Castagnoli P, Layton B, Beutler B. Defective LPS signaling in C3H/HeJ and C57BL/10 Sccr mice: mutations in Tr 4 gene. Science 1998; 282:2085–2088.

[52] Rosenfeld V, Benfeldt E, Valerius NH, Paerregaard A, Michaesen KF. Effect of probiotics on gastrointestinal symptoms and small intestinal permeability in children with atopic dermatitis. J Pediatr 2004; 145:612–616

[53] Wilson MS, Tayor MD, Balic A, Finney CA, Lamb JR, Maizels RM. Suppression of allergic airway inflammation by helminth induced regulatory T cells. J Exp Med 2005; 202:1199–1212.

[54] Cario E. Bacterial interactions with cells of the intestinal mucosa: toll like receptors and NOD 2. Gut 2005; 54:1182–1193

[55] Veckman V, Mieltinen M, Matikainen S, Lande R, Giacomini E, Coccia EM, Julkunen I. Lactobacilli and Streptococci induce inflammatory chemokine production in human macrophages that stimulate Th1 cell chemotaxis. J Leuko Biol 2003; 74(3):395–402.

[56] Turnbaugh PJ, Ley RE, Mahowald MA, Magrini V, Mardis ER, Gordon JI. An obesity associated gut microbiome with increased capacity for energy harvest. Nature 2006; 444(7122):1027–1031.

[57] Fei N, Zhao L. An opportunistic pathogen isolated from the gut of an obese human causes obesity in germfree mice. Int Soc Microb Ecol 2012; 12:1–5.

[58] Can PD, Delzenne NM, Amar J, Burcelin R. Role of gut microflora in the development of obesity and insulin resistance following high fat diet feeding. Pathol Biol 2008; 56(5): 305–309.

[59] Bajjer M, Seeley RJ. Physiology: obesity and gut flora. Nature 2006; 444:1009–1010.

[60] Ridaura VK, Faith JJ, Rey FE, Cheng J, Duncan AE, Kau AL, Griffin NW, Lombard V, Henrissat B, Bain JR, Muehlbauer MJ, Ilkayeva O, Semenkovich CF, Funai K, Hayashi DK, Lyle BJ, Martini MC, Ursell LK, Clemente JC, Van Treuren W, Walters WA, Knight R, Newgard CB, Heath AC, Gordon JI. Gut microbiota from twins discordant for obesity modulate metabolism in mice. Science 2013; 341(6150):1241214

[61] Bäckhed F, Ding H, Wang T, Hooper LV, Koh GY, Nagy A, Semenkovich CF, Gordon JI. The gut microbiota as an environmental factor that regulates fat storage. Proc Natl Acad Sci USA 2004;104:15718–15723.

[62] Turn bough PJ, Ley RE, Mahowald MA, Magvini V, Mardis ER, Gordon JI. An obesity associated gut microbiome with increased capacity for energy harvest. Nature 2006; 444:1027–1031.

[63] Cani PD, Amar J, Iglesias MA, Poggi M, Knauf C, Bastelica D, Neyrinck AM, Fava F, Tuohy KM, Chabo C, Waget A, Delmée E, Cousin B, Sulpice T, Chamontin B, Ferrières J, Tanti JF, Gibson GR, Casteilla L, Delzenne NM, Alessi MC, Burcelin R. Metabolic endotoxemia initiates obesity and insulin resistance. Diabetes 2007; 56:1761–1772.

[64] Creely SJ, McTernan PG, Kusminski CM, Fisher FM, Da Silva NF, Khanolkar M, Evans M, Harte AL, Kumar S. Lipopolysaccharide activates an innate immune system response in human adipose tissue in obesity and type 2 diabetes. Am J Physiol Endocrinol Metab 2007; 292:E740–E747.

[65] Carvalho BM, Saad MJ. Influence of gut microbiota on subclinical inflammation and insulin resistance. Mediators Inflamm,20132;2013(13):986734, http/doi 10.1155//2013/986734.

[66] Arumugam M, Raes J, Pelletier E, Le Paslier D, Yamada T, Mende DR, Fernandes GR, Tap J, Bruls T, Batto JM, Bertalan M, Borruel N, Casellas F, Fernandez L, Gautier L, Hansen T, Hattori M, Hayashi T, Kleerebezem M, Kurokawa K, Leclerc M, Levenez F, Manichanh C, Nielsen HB, Nielsen T, Pons N, Poulain J, Qin J, Sicheritz-Ponten T, Tims

http://dx.doi.org/10.5772/65073

S, Torrents D, Ugarte E, Zoetendal EG, Wang J, Guarner F, Pedersen O, de Vos WM, Brunak S, Doré J; MetaHIT Consortium, Antolín M, Artiguenave F, Blottiere HM, Almeida M, Brechot C, Cara C, Chervaux C, Cultrone A, Delorme C, Denariaz G, Dervyn R, Foerstner KU, Friss C, van de Guchte M, Guedon E, Haimet F, Huber W, van Hylckama-Vlieg J, Jamet A, Juste C, Kaci G, Knol J, Lakhdari O, Layec S, Le Roux K, Maguin E, Mérieux A, Melo Minardi R, M'rini C, Muller J, Oozeer R, Parkhill J, Renault P, Rescigno M, Sanchez N, Sunagawa S, Torrejon A, Turner K, Vandemeulebrouck G, Varela E, Winogradsky Y, Zeller G, Weissenbach J, Ehrlich SD, Bork P. Enterotypes of the human gut microbiome. Nature 2011; 43:174–180.